D0931421

WALKER'S MANLY EXERCISES

WALKER'S MANLY EXERCISES

CONTAINING

Walking, Running, Leaping, Vaulting, Climbing, Skating, Swimming

AND OTHER MANLY SPORTS

BY DONALD WALKER

MICHAEL JOSEPH
AN IMPRINT OF
PENGUIN BOOKS

MICHAEL JOSEPH

UK | USA | Canada | Ireland | Australia
India | New Zealand | South Africa

Michael Joseph is part of the Penguin Random House group of companies
whose addresses can be found at global.penguinrandomhouse.com

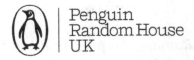

First published by Thomas Hurst 1834
This edition published by Michael Joseph 2018
001

Set in New Baskerville ITC Pro and Bulmer MT Pro
Typeset by Jouve (UK), Milton Keynes
Printed in Great Britain by Clays Ltd, St Ives plc

A CIP catalogue record for this book is available from the British Library

HARDBACK ISBN: 978-0-241-34915-1

www.greenpenguin.co.uk

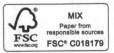

CONTENTS

IMPORTANCE OF PHYSICAL EXERCISES

LOCOMOTIVE EXERCISES

AQUATIC EXERCISES

LIST OF PLATES

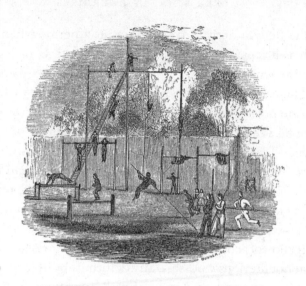

IMPORTANCE OF PHYSICAL EXERCISES

EDUCATION may be divided into two parts, physical and mental. Of the former, EXERCISES or GYMNASTICS are the most extensive and the earliest portion.

Their extent is learnt by an enumeration of them, viz. Walking, Running, Leaping, Vaulting, Pole-leaping, Balancing, Carrying, Climbing, Skating, and Swimming.

The object of these Exercises is to strengthen the muscular system, by subjecting it to a regular process of training, and to teach the means of employing it most advantageously. The expediency of their early acquisition is rendered evident by the first tendency of youth being directed to them, by the rapid progress made in them, and by the delight derived from them, at a period when the body is incapable, with real or solid advantage, of higher acquirements.

Their general utility will be questioned only by those who are not aware that the health and vigour of all the bodily organs depend on the proportioned exercise of each. In active exertion, the member exercised swells with the more frequent and more copious flow of blood, and heat is developed in it with greater abundance; and if we repeat the same motions many times after intervals of repose, all the muscles exercised become permanently developed; a perfection of action ensues in the member exercised, which it did not previously possess, any deformity by which it is affected is corrected, and strength and activity are acquired. That man, therefore, gains the most strength who engages in muscular exercises that require the application of much power, but which are sufficiently separated by intervals of repose.

It must be remembered, however, that, in exercising particular muscles only, the others become weak. The strength of Marshal Saxe was sufficiently great to stop a chariot drawn at speed by four horses, by merely seizing the wheel: he bent pieces of silver with his fingers, made them into boats as he would with paper, and presented them to the ladies. Count Orloff, a Russian general, broke the shoe of a carriage horse in the same manner; and there are innumerable examples of similar feats of extraordinary strength.

Active exercises, at the same time, confer beauty of form; and they even contribute to impart an elegant air and graceful manners. If the exercise of a limb be continued for some time, the member swells, a painful sensation is experienced, which is termed lassitude, and a difficulty of contraction, which is the result of it. If the motion has been excessive, and the organic elements in the member have been acted upon beyond all physiological laws, inflammation would take place, and its functions be performed with great difficulty, if at all.

Such are the effects of exercise on the locomotive system, to all the functions of animated beings, so long as they are exercised with moderation, equality, and at due intervals, working for their own preservation. Of course, the general effect of active exercises is marked in proportion to the number of parts that share in the motion, or are brought into energetic action. In general exercise, the increase of organic action is not confined solely to the parts which are the seat of muscular contraction, but is repeated throughout all parts of the economy, and influences all the functions.

Thus, as to the vital or nutritive system, exercises taken when digestion is not going on, excite the digestive faculty: taken during its progress, they disorder that function. The arterial and venous circulations become more rapid by active exercise, which concludes by giving greater force to the tissue of the heart. It is the same with respiration and calorification. The same takes place with regard to nutrition, a function which exercise increases, not only in the muscles in movement, as we have just seen, but also in the bones, ligaments, vessels, and nerves.

By inducing cutaneous exhalation, it promotes the expulsion of injurious agents, produces a fresh colour in persons who may have become pale through a sedentary life, and, to a certain extent, renders the human constitution, by means of habit, proof against the action of surrounding objects. The local effects of excessive action, or those which take place in the members themselves, are, as before observed, inflammation of the muscles, rheumatism, like that arising from cold, and inflammation of the serous articular membranes. The general effects of excessive exercise may, in the same manner as all physical and moral stimulants, exhaust the vital faculties too quickly, communicate too much rigidity to the fibres, render the vessels varicose, bring on chronic rheumatism, destroy the freshness of the skin, blight the flower of youth, and produce old age and death before the time ordained by nature.

Ancient writers inform us that it was a rare thing to meet with athletes, who, having signalized themselves from their earliest youth in gymnastic combats, were of so excellent a constitution as to be able, when they had reached a more advanced age, to acquire the same honours in contending for the prize with grown men. Aristotle assures us, that amongst the conquerors in the Olympic Games, not more than two or three at the most could be found to whom nature had granted such an advantage.

In relation to the mental or thinking system, 'every movement,' says Cabanis, 'becomes in its turn the principle or occasion of new impressions, of which the frequent repetition and the varied character must increase more and more the circle of our judgments, or tend unceasingly to rectify them. It hence follows that labour, giving to this word the most general signification, cannot but have an influence infinitely useful on the habits of the understanding, and consequently also on those of the will.' This argument is evidently applicable to varied exercise. On the contrary, 'the great division of labour, so favourable to the perfecting of the arts, contracts more and more the understanding of workmen.' Exercises, moreover, inspire confidence in difficult situations, and suggest resources in danger. Their consequent influence upon the moral conduct of man is such, that, by a courage which is well founded, because it springs from a perfect knowledge of his own powers, he is often enabled to render the most important services to others.

Although the direct effect of exercise is not only to confer power on the muscular and other organs, but to multiply external impressions, and to occupy with them all the senses at once; still minds thus disposed, in general occupy themselves rather with objects of imagination and sentiment, than with those which demand more complicated operation. The sense of muscular power impresses determinations which, carrying man perpetually out of himself, scarcely permit him to dwell upon impressions transmitted to his brain. The only action of that organ, during these exercises, seems to be limited to ordering the movements.

Hence, exercise, especially taken in the open air, amidst new and varied objects of sight, is not favourable to reflection – to labours which demand the assemblage and concentration of all the powers of the mind. It is, on the contrary, in the absence of external impressions, that we become more capable of seizing many relations, and of following a long train of purely abstract reasoning. As life spent chiefly in active muscular exercises would leave in a state of repose those central organs that are subservient to the moral qualities and intellectual faculties, I agree with Seneca and Camper, in proscribing all such exercises, or such degrees of exercise, as would exhaust the mind, and render man incapable of aptitude in science, polite literature, and art.

The cultivation of bodily strength, in preference to everything else, would establish only the right of the strongest, as it is found to exist in the origin of society. To cultivate the faculties of the mind exclusively, would produce only the weakness of sentiment or excess of passion. There is, for every individual, a means of making all these dispositions act in harmony; and the due blending of physical and moral education alone can produce it. Let it be remembered that young persons will much more easily be withdrawn from the application they ought to pay to the study of the sciences, by insipid recreations and trifling games, than by the fatiguing exercises necessary for their development and the preservation of their health, which, however, habit soon renders easy and delightful. To what vices do not a sedentary life and the practice of gaming give rise? – whilst well-regulated exercises excite ambition to excel, and energy in the performance of every duty.

The philosophers of antiquity, such as Aristotle and Plato, regarded gymnastic exercises as of vast importance, and considered a state defective and badly organized where these exercises were not instituted. Colleges, called Gymnasia, were therefore established everywhere, and superintended by distinguished masters. Accordingly, the illustrious men of the Grecian and Roman republics, even those who shone in literature and the fine arts, received the same physical education. The gymnastic exercises which are here recommended are not intended to produce athletes, but to strengthen the human constitution. One exercise gives solidity, another address; and we may even say that the various kinds of exercise are sometimes opposed to each other. The strongest peasant is far from being the best runner; and the most vigorous dancer would probably be deficient in strength. There is, however, a mean to be found in the disposition of every individual to preserve both skill and strength, and this is what ought to be sought. For this purpose, it will be sufficient for young persons to practise a few hours every day, sometimes at one exercise, and sometimes at another.

GENERAL DIRECTIONS

IT only remains for us to give a few directions as to the time, place, and circumstances of exercise. The best time for the elementary exercises is when the air is cool, as, even in summer, it is early in the morning, or after the sun has declined; and they should never immediately follow a meal. The best place for these elementary exercises is a smooth patch of grass, or a firm, sandy sea-beach. Chasms, stones, and stakes, are always dangerous. At the commencement, the coat and all unnecessary clothes should be laid aside; and all hard or sharp things should be taken from the pockets of the remaining dress. A very light covering on the head, as a straw hat, is best; the shirt-collar should be open, the breast being either exposed or thinly covered; the waistband of the trousers should not be tight, and the boots or shoes should have no iron about them.

As sudden transitions are always bad, exercise should

begin gently, and should terminate in the same manner. The left hand and arm being commonly weaker than the right, they should be exercised till they become as strong. This custom is advantageous, not only for all military and mechanical gymnastic exercises, but also for all their operations. Being cooled too quickly is injurious. Therefore, drinking when very hot, or lying down on the cold ground, should be carefully avoided. No exertion should be carried to excess, as that only exhausts and enfeebles the body. Therefore, whenever the gymnast feels tired, or falls behind his usual mark, he should resume his clothes, and walk home. The moment exercise is finished, the clothes should always be put on, and the usual precautions adopted to prevent taking cold.

The necessary fittings-up of an exercising ground are a leaping stand, a vaulting horse, a balancing bar, a climbing stand, with ladders, poles, and ropes, which may be seen united as simply and economically as possible, in a subsequent sketch (Plate XVIII CLIMBING).

In most exercises, a belt or cincture is of utility; and it seems, in all ages, to have been naturally employed. The weakest savage, who could not follow others in the course without panting, would find, by placing his hand over his abdomen, and supporting the liver and other organs which descend into that cavity, that he was aided in running, and breathed more easily; and thence he would make for himself a belt. United in societies, men would still preserve their belt, though it might not seem particularly advantageous, except to those whose active mode of life approached a primitive state, such as travellers, couriers, and porters.

The Greeks put on their belts before they commenced

wrestling; and many physicians, both ancient and modern, recommend the use of belts, as being to the whole of the body, and to the parts over which they are placed, what the exterior sheaths or aponeuroses are to the muscles – bands which embrace and keep firm the parts over which they are placed. The common belt has leathern straps, and buckles to fasten it, an iron ring and a pocket. A double cincture for wrestling forms a very strong girth, which is put on by pupils who are very strong, when they wrestle. These belts may be made of different sizes, for youths of different ages: of five or six inches for tall youths and men, and of eight or ten inches for wrestlers. Their length is in proportion to the size of the person who uses them. These belts are very useful in strengthening the abdominal region in running and leaping. Riders, also, should furnish themselves with belts before getting on horseback, to prevent too violent motion of the viscera of the abdomen, and the disorders which may result from it. The use, indeed, of belts will by degrees prove their utility, and they will probably be worn even externally, without reference to physical exercises. They deserve this the more, because they give an air of lightness and elegance to the shape, and develop the chest.

The most useful thing in existence is dangerous, if improperly applied. In very young persons, the chest and abdomen have been compressed by fastening the belt too tight, or making it too wide; and disorders of digestion and respiration have consequently been caused by pushing in the false ribs. This is an imprudence that should be avoided. If the belt be too low, it may press too much on the lower part of the belly; if too high, it may disorder the chest. It must therefore be placed on the loins, so as to pass over the navel; and, as said before, it must not be too tight. Having given these ideas of the utility of belts, and the manner of using them, it remains only to explain the triple use of those adopted for exercises: Firstly, they fulfill, by their size and other circumstances, all the conditions which render them useful; Secondly, a pocket serves to enclose the articles that may be wanted, according to the class of exercises being performed; Thirdly, an iron ring is intended to suspend, by means of hooks, any thing we wish to carry, so as to leave the hands at liberty.

TRAINING

THIS is important in relation to various exercises to be described. The art of training for athletic exercises, or labourious exertions, consists in purifying the body and strengthening its powers, by certain processes, which are now to be described. The advantages of it, however, are not confined to pedestrians, wrestlers, or pugilists; they extend to everyone: for, were training generally introduced, instead of medicine, for the prevention and cure of diseases, its beneficial consequences would assuredly prolong life, and promote its happiness. Every physiologist knows that all the parts which compose the human body – solids as well as liquids – are successively absorbed and deposited. Hence ensues a perpetual renovation of them, regulated by the nature of our food and general habits. The health of all the parts, and the soundness of their structure, depend on this perpetual absorption and renovation. Now, nothing works as effectively as exercise to excite at once absorption and secretion. It accordingly promotes all the vital functions without hurrying them, renovates all the parts, and preserves them apt and fit for their offices.

It follows, then, that health, vigour, and activity, chiefly depend upon exercise and regimen; or, in other words, upon the observance of those rules which constitute the theory of training. The effect has accordingly corresponded with the cause assigned in this view of the subject, in every instance where it has been adopted; and, although not commonly resorted to as the means of restoring invalids to health, there is every reason to believe that it would prove effectual in curing many obstinate diseases, such as bilious complaints, obesity, gout, and rheumatism.

The ancients entertained this opinion. They were, says a popular writer on medicine, by no means unacquainted with or inattentive to these instruments of medicine, although modern practitioners appear to have no idea of removing disease, or restoring health, but by pouring drugs into the stomach. Heroditus is said to have been the first who applied the exercises and regimen of the Gymnasium to the removal of disease, or the maintenance of health. Among the Romans, Asclepiades carried this so far, that he is said, by Celsus, almost to have banished the use of internal remedies from his practice. He was the inventor of various modes of exercise and gestation in Rome. In his own person, he afforded an excellent example of the wisdom of his rules, and the propriety of his regimen. Pliny tells us that, in early life, he made a public profession, that he would agree to forfeit all pretensions to the name of a physician, should he ever suffer from sickness, or die but of old age; and, what is extraordinary, he fulfilled his promise, for he lived upwards of a century, and at last was killed by a fall down stairs.

As to the locomotive system, modern experience sufficiently proves that exercise is the most powerful strengthener of the muscles, and of every part on which activity depends. In its operation on the vital system, training always appears to benefit the state of the lungs. Indeed, one of its most striking effects is to improve the wind: that is, to enable a man to draw a larger inspiration, and to hold his breath longer. As to the intellectual system, Sir J. Sinclair observes that, by training, the mental faculties are also improved; the attention being more ready, and the perception more acute, owing probably to the clearness of the stomach, and better digestion.

It must, therefore, be admitted, that the most beneficial consequences to general health arise from training. The simplicity of the rules for it is assuredly a great recommendation to a trial of the experiment. The whole process may be resolved into the following principles: Firstly, the evacuating, which cleanses the stomach and intestines; Secondly, the sweating, which takes off the superfluities of fat and humours; Thirdly, the daily course of exercise, which improves the wind and strengthens the muscles; and, lastly, the regimen, which nourishes and invigorates the body. To those who are to engage in corporeal exercises beyond their ordinary powers, it is indispensably necessary. Pedestrians, therefore, who are matched either against others or against time, and pugilists who engage to fight, must undergo the training process before they contend. The issue of the contest, if their powers be nearly equal, will, in a great measure, depend upon their relative condition, as effected by training, at the hour of trial.

Training was known to the ancients, who paid much attention to the means of augmenting corporeal vigour and activity. Accordingly, among the Greeks and Romans, certain rules of exercise and regimen were prescribed to the candidates for gymnastic celebrity. We are assured that, among the Greeks, previously to the solemn contests at the public games, the strictest temperance, sobriety, and regularity in living, were indispensably requisite. The candidates were, at the same time, subjected to daily exercise in the Gymnasium, which continued during ten months, and which, with the prescribed regimen, constituted the preparatory training adopted by the athletae of Greece. Among the Romans, the exercises of the palaestra degenerated from the rank of a liberal art, and became a profession, which was embraced only by the lowest of mankind; the exhibitions of the gladiators being bloody and ferocious spectacles, which evinced the barbarous taste of the people. The combatants, however, were regularly trained by proper exercise, and a strict observance of regimen. Pure and salubrious air was deemed a chief requisite. Accordingly, the principal schools of their athletae were established at Capua and Ravenna, the most healthy places in Italy; and previous to entering on this regimen, the men were subjected to the evacuating process, by means of emetics, which they preferred to purgatives.

In the more early stages of training, their diet consisted of dried figs, new cheese, and boiled grain. Afterwards animal food was introduced as a part of the athletic regimen, and pork was preferred to any other. Galen, indeed, asserts that pork contains more real nutriment than flesh of any other kind, which is used as food by man. This fact, he adds, is decidedly proved by the example of the athletae, who, if they live but for one day on any other kind of food, find their vigour manifestly impaired the next. The preference given to pork by the ancients, however, does not correspond with the practice of modern trainers, who entirely reject it; but in the manner of preparing the food, they exactly agree – roasting or broiling being by both preferred to boiling, and bread unfermented to that prepared by leaven. A very small quantity of liquid was allowed to the athletae, and this was principally water. They exercised in the open air, and became familiarized by habit to every change of the weather, the vicissitudes of which soon ceased to affect them.

To exercise their patience, and accustom them to bear pain without flinching, they were occasionally flogged on the back with the branches of a kind of rhododendron, till the blood flowed. By diminishing the quantity of the circulating liquid, this rough kind of cupping was also considered salutary! as obviating the tendency to plethora or redundancy of blood, to which they were peculiarly liable – a proof, if true, of the nourishing qualities of their food.

When the daily exercises of the athletae were finished, they were refreshed by immersion in a tepid bath, where the perspiration and sordes – scurf, pustules, or filthy adhesions – were carefully removed from the surface of the body by the use of the strygil.[1] The skin was then diligently rubbed dry, and again anointed with oil. If thirsty, they were

---

1. For this instrument, rough coarse clothes are adopted, but not with advantage.

permitted to drink a small quantity of warm water. They then took their principal repast, after which they used no more exercise that day. They occasionally also went into the cold bath in the morning. They were permitted to sleep as many hours as they chose; and great increase of vigour, as well as of bulk, was supposed to be derived from long-continued and sound repose.[2] The sexual intercourse was strictly prohibited.

The manner of training among the ancients bears some resemblance to that practised by the moderns. Perhaps it is because their mode of living and general habits were somewhat different from those of the present age, that a difference of treatment is now required to produce the same effects. The great object of training for running or boxing matches, is to increase the muscular strength, and to improve the free action of the lungs, or wind, of the person subjected to the process. Seeing that the human body is so capable of being altered and renovated, it is not surprising that the art of training should be carried to a degree of perfection almost incredible; and that, by certain processes, the muscular power, the breath (or wind), and the courage of man, should be so greatly improved as to enable him to perform the most severe or labourious undertakings.

That such effects have been produced is unquestionable: they are fully exemplified in the astonishing exploits of our most celebrated pedestrians and pugilists, which are the infallible results of such preparatory discipline. The

2. Little sleep is now prescribed; but its quantity should depend upon circumstances of fatigue, &c.

skilful trainer attends to the state of the bowels, the lungs, and the skin; and he uses such means as will reduce the fat, and at the same time invigorate the muscular fibre. The patient is purged by drastic medicines; he is sweated by walking under a load of clothes, and by lying between feather beds; and his limbs are roughly rubbed. His diet is beef or mutton; his drink strong ale. He is gradually inured to exercise, by repeated trials in walking and running. By extenuating the fat, emptying the cellular substance, hardening the muscular fibre, and improving the breath, a man of the ordinary frame may be made to fight for one hour, with the utmost exertion of strength and courage, or to go over one hundred miles in twenty-four hours.

The most effectual process for training appears to be that practised by Captain Barclay, which has not only been sanctioned by professional men, but has met with the unqualified approbation of amateurs. We are here, therefore, almost entirely indebted to it for details. According to this method, the pedestrian, who may be supposed in tolerable condition, enters upon his training with a regular course of physic, which consists of three doses. Glauber's salts are generally preferred; and from one ounce and a half to two ounces are taken each time, with an interval of four days between each dose. After having gone through the course of physic, he commences his regular exercise, which is gradually increased as he proceeds in the training.

When the object in view is the accomplishment of a pedestrian match, his regular exercise may be from twenty to twenty-four miles a day. He must rise at five in the morning, run half a mile at the top of his speed up-hill, and then walk six miles at a moderate pace, coming in about seven to breakfast, which should consist of beef-steaks or mutton-chops under-done, with stale bread and old beer. After breakfast, he must again walk six miles at a moderate pace, and at twelve lie down in bed, without his clothes, for half an hour. On getting up, he must walk four miles, and return by four to dinner, which should also be beefsteaks or mutton-chops, with bread and beer, as at breakfast. Immediately after dinner, he must resume his exercise, by running half a mile at the top of his speed, and walking six miles at a moderate pace. He takes no more exercise for that day, but retires to bed about eight; and next morning he proceeds in the same manner.

Animal diet, it will be observed, is, according to this system, alone prescribed, and beef and mutton are preferred. All fat and greasy substances are prohibited, as they induce bile, and consequently injure the stomach. The lean of meat contains more nourishment than the fat; and in every case, the most substantial food is preferable to any other kind. Fresh meat is the most wholesome and nourishing. Salt, spiceries, and all kinds of seasonings, with the exception of vinegar, are prohibited. The lean, then, of fat beef cooked in steaks, with very little salt, is the best; and it should be rather under-done than otherwise. Mutton, being reckoned easy of digestion, may be occasionally given, to vary the diet and gratify the taste. The legs of fowls are also esteemed.

It is preferable to have the meat broiled, as much of its nutritive quality is lost by roasting or boiling. It ought to be dressed so as to remain tender and juicy; for it is by these means that it will be easily digested, and afford most nourishment. Biscuit and stale bread are the only preparations of vegetable matter which are permitted to be given; and everything inducing flatulency must be carefully avoided. In general, the quantity of aliment is not limited by the trainer, but left entirely to the discretion of the pedestrian, whose appetite should regulate him in this respect.

With respect to liquors, they must be always taken cold; and home-brewed beer, old, but not bottled, is the best. A little red wine, however, may be given to those who are not fond of malt liquor; but never more than half a pint after dinner. It is an established rule to avoid liquids as much as possible; and no more liquor of any kind is allowed to be taken than is requisite to quench the thirst.

After having gone on in this regular course for three or four weeks, the pedestrian must take a four mile-sweat, which is produced by running four miles in flannel, at the top of his speed. Immediately on returning, a hot liquor is prescribed, in order to promote the perspiration; and of this he must drink one English pint. It is termed the sweating liquor, and is composed of one ounce of carraway seed, half an ounce of coriander seed, one ounce of root-liquorice, and half an ounce of sugar-candy, mixed with two bottles of cider, and boiled down to one-half. He is then put to bed in his flannels, and, being covered with six or eight pair of blankets, and a feather bed, must remain in this state from twenty-five to thirty minutes, when he is taken out, and rubbed perfectly dry. Being then well wrapt in his great-coat, he walks out gently for two miles, and returns to breakfast, which, on such occasions, should consist of a roasted fowl. He afterwards proceeds with his usual exercise.

These sweats are continued weekly, till within a few

days of the performance of the match; or, in other words, he must undergo three or four of these operations. If the stomach of the pedestrian be foul, an emetic or two must be given about a week before the conclusion of the training. He is now supposed to be in the highest condition.

Besides his usual or regular exercise, a person under training ought to employ himself, in the intervals, in every kind of exertion which tends to activity, such as golf, cricket, bowls, throwing quoits, &c., so that, during the whole day, both body and mind may be constantly occupied. Although the chief parts of the system depend upon sweating, exercise, and feeding, yet the object to be obtained by the pedestrian would be defeated, if these were not adjusted each to the other, and to his constitution. The trainer, before he proceeds to apply his theory, should make himself acquainted with the constitution and habits of his patient, that he may be able to judge how far he can, with safety, carry on the different parts of the process. The nature of the patient's disposition should also be known, that every cause of irritation may be avoided; for, as it requires great patience and perseverance to undergo training, every expedient to soothe and encourage the mind should be adopted.

The skilful trainer will, moreover, constantly study the progress of his art, by observing the effect of its processes, separately and in combination. If a man retain his health and spirits during the process, improve in wind, and increase in strength, it is certain that the object aimed at will be obtained; but, if otherwise, it is to be apprehended that some defect exists, through the unskilfulness or mismanagement of the trainer, which ought instantly to be remedied by such alterations as the circumstances of the case may demand. It is evident, therefore, that in many instances the trainer must be guided by his judgment, and that no fixed rules of management can, with absolute certainty, be depended upon, for producing an invariable and determinate result. In general, however, it may be calculated, that the known rules are adequate to the purpose, if the pedestrian strictly adhere to them, and the trainer bestow a moderate degree of attention to his state and condition during the progress of training.

It is impossible to fix any precise period for the completion of the training process, as it depends upon the previous condition of the pedestrian; but from two to three months, in most cases, will be sufficient, especially if he be in tolerable condition at the commencement, and possessed of sufficient perseverance and courage to submit cheerfully to the privations and hardships to which he must unavoidably be subjected. The criterion by which it may be known whether a man is in good condition – or, what is the same thing, whether he has been properly trained – is the state of the skin, which becomes smooth, elastic, and well-coloured or transparent. The flesh is also firm; and the person trained feels himself light, and full of spirits. In the progress of the training, his condition may also be ascertained by the effect of the sweats, which cease to reduce his weight; and by the manner in which he performs one mile at the top of his speed. It is as difficult to run a mile at the top of one's speed as to walk a hundred; and therefore, if he perform this short distance well, it may be concluded that his condition is perfect, or that he has derived all the advantages which can possibly result from the training process.

A few words may be here added on the comparative strength of different races of men. In order to procure some exact results on this point, Peron took with him on his voyage an instrument called a dynamometer, so constructed as to indicate on a dial-plate the relative force of individuals submitted to experiment. He directed his attention to the strength of the arms and of the loins, making trial with several individuals of each of the races among whom he then was, viz. twelve natives of Van Diemen's Land, seventeen of New Holland, fifty-six of the Island of Timor, seventeen Frenchmen belonging to the expedition, and fourteen Englishmen in the colony of New South Wales. The following numbers express the mean result in each case, but all the details are given in a tabular form in the original:

	Strength of the Arms Kilogrammes	Strength of the Loins Myriagrammes
1. Van Diemen's Land · ·	50.6	10.1
2. New Holland · · ·	50.8	10.2
3. Timor · · · · ·	58.7	11.6
4. French · · · · ·	69.2	15.2
5. English · · · ·	71.4	16.3

The highest numbers in the first and second class were, respectively, 60 and 62; the lowest in the English trials 63, and the highest 83, for the strength of the arms. In the power of the loins, the highest among the New Hollanders was 13; the lowest of the English 12.7, and the highest 21.3. 'These results,' observes Mr Lawrence, 'offer the best answer to declamations on the degeneracy of civilized man. The attribute of superior physical strength, so boldly assumed by the eulogists of the savage state, has never been questioned or doubted. Although we have been consoled for this supposed inferiority by an enumeration of the many precious benefits derived from civilization, it has always been felt as a somewhat degrading disadvantage. Bodily strength is a concomitant of good health, which is produced and supported by a regular supply of wholesome and nutritious food, and by active occupation. The industrious and well-fed middle classes of a civilized community may, therefore, be reasonably expected to surpass, in this endowment, the miserable savages, who are never well-fed, and too frequently depressed by absolute want and all other privations.'

POSITION

BEFORE entering into a detail of exercises, it is necessary to attend to what is termed position. A standing position is the action by which we keep ourselves up. Indeed, this state, in which the body appears in repose, is itself an exercise, for it consists in a continued effort of many muscles; and the explanation we shall give of it will much facilitate that of walking.

Everyone has observed that during sleep, or a fainting fit, the head inclines forward and falls upon the breast. In this case, it is in accordance with the laws of gravity; for the head, resting upon the vertebrae which support it at a point of its basis which is nearer the posterior than anterior part, cannot remain in an upright position in standing, except by an effort of the muscles at the back of the neck: it is the cessation of this effort that causes it to fall forward. The body also is unable to remain straight without fatigue. The vertebral column being placed behind, all the viscera or parts contained by the chest and belly are suspended in front of it, and would force it to bend forward unless strong muscular fibres held it back. A proof of this may be seen in pregnant and dropsical women, who are compelled, in consequence of the anterior part of the body being heavier than usual, to keep the vertebral column more fixed, and even thrown backward. The same observation may be made with regard to the pelvis basin, or lowest part of the trunk, which by its conformation would bend upon the thighs, if not kept back by the great mass of muscular fibres that form the hips. In front of the thighs, again, are the muscles which, by keeping the kneepan in position, are the means of preventing the leg from bending. Lastly, the muscles forming the calves, by contracting, are the means of preventing the leg from bending upon the foot.

Such is the general mechanism of the standing position. It is, therefore, as we observed, a concurrence of efforts: almost all the extending muscles are in a state of contraction all the time that this position is maintained, and the consequence is, a fatigue which cannot be endured for any great length of time. Hence we see persons in a standing position rest the weight of their body, first on one foot, then on another, for the purpose of procuring momentary ease to certain muscles. For this reason, also, standing still is more fatiguing than walking, in which the muscles are alternately contracted and extended.

A question of importance on this subject is, what position of the feet affords the greatest solidity in standing? We will not enter into detail of the numerous controversies by which some have defended or repudiated the position with the toes turned forward or outward: it will be sufficient to state the fact, that the larger the base of support, the firmer and more solid will the position be, and to adopt, as a *fundamental* one, the military position, which has been found practically the best by those who have nothing else to do but to walk. The equal squareness of the shoulders and body to the front, is the first great principle of position. The heels must be in a line, and closed; the knees straight; the toes turned out, with the feet forming an angle of sixty degrees; the arms hanging close to the body; the elbows turned in, and close to the sides; the hands open to the front, with the view of preserving the elbow in the position above described; the little fingers lightly touching the clothing of the limbs, with the thumb close to the forefinger; the belly rather drawn in, and the breast advanced, but without constraint; the body upright, but inclining forward, so that the weight of it may principally bear upon the fore part of the feet; the head erect, and the eyes straight to the front (as in Plate I. *fig.* 1).

To these brief directions I must add that, in standing, the whole figure should be in such a position that the ear, shoulder, haunch, knee, and ankle are all in a line; that it must be stretched as much as possible, by raising the back of the head, drawing in the chin, straightening the spine, rising on the hips, and extending the legs; that the object of keeping the back thus straight is to allow of standing longer without fatigue; that it is important to expand the chest, and to throw the shoulders back, with the shoulder-blades, or scapulae, quite flat behind; and that though, in military instructions, the body is thus inclined forward in standing without arms, yet when these are assumed, the body is immediately thrown about two inches backward, into a nearly perpendicular position. This position, therefore, will be modified in walking, and especially in ordinary walking; but it is an excellent fundamental position, and it cannot be too accurately acquired.

This is the amount of the drill-sergeant's instructions as to position, though this last part is omitted in the Manual describing the Field Exercise and Evolutions of the Army.

EXTENSION MOTIONS

In order to supple the figure, open the chest, and give freedom to the muscles, the first three movements of the extension motions, as laid down for the sword exercise, are ordered to be practised. It is, indeed, observed that too many methods cannot be used to improve the carriage, and banish a rustic air; but that the greatest care must be taken not to throw the body backward instead of forward, as being contrary to every true principle of movement. I accordingly here introduce these extension motions, adding the fourth and fifth, and prefixing to each the respective word of command, in order that they may be the more distinctly and accurately executed.

Attention. The body is to be erect, the heels close together, and the hands hanging down on each side.

First Extension Motion. This serves as a caution, and the motions tend to expand the chest, raise the head, throw back the shoulders, and strengthen the muscles of the back.

PLATE I

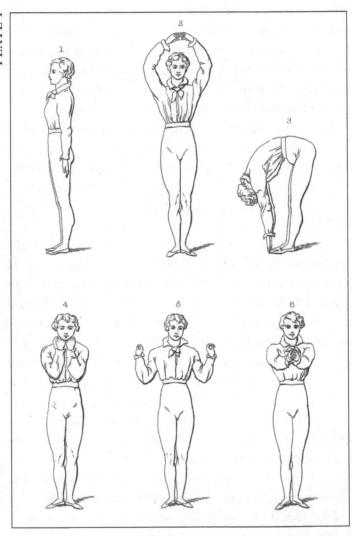

POSITION – EXTENSION MOTIONS

One. Bring the hands and arms to the front, the fingers lightly touching at the points, and the nails downward; then raise them in a circular direction well above the head, the ends of the fingers still touching, the thumbs pointing to the rear, the elbows pressed back, and shoulders kept down (Plate I. *fig.* 2).

Two. Separate and extend the arms and fingers, forcing them obliquely back, till they come extended on a line with the shoulders; and as they fall gradually from thence to the original position of Attention, endeavour, as much as possible, to elevate the neck and chest. These two motions should be frequently practised, with the head turned as much as possible to the right or left, and the body kept square to the front: this tends very materially to supple the neck, &c.

Three. Turn the palms of the hands to the front, pressing back the thumbs with the arms extended, and raise them to the rear, till they meet above the head; the fingers pointing upward, with the ends of the thumbs touching.

Four. Keep the arms and knees straight, and bend over from the hips till the hands touch the feet, the head being brought down in the same direction (Plate I. *fig.* 3).

Five. With the arms flexible and easy from the shoulders, raise the body gradually, so as to resume the position of Attention.

The whole should be done very gradually, so as to feel the exertion of the muscles throughout. To these extension motions, drill-sergeants, in their instructions, add the following:

One. The forearms are bent upon the arms upward and towards the body, having the elbows depressed, the shut hands touching on the little-finger sides, and the knuckles upward, the latter being raised as high as the chin, and at the distance of about a foot before it (Plate I. *fig.* 4).

Two. While the arms are thrown forcibly backward, the forearms are as much as possible bent upon the arms, and the palmar sides of the wrists are turned forward and outward (Plate I. *fig.* 5). The two motions are to be repeatedly and rather quickly performed. A modification of the same movement is performed as a separate extension motion, but may be given in continuation, with the numbers following these, as words of command.

Three. The arms are extended at full length in front, on a level with the shoulder, the palms of the hands in contact (Plate I. *fig.* 6).

Four. Thus extended, and the palms retaining their vertical position, the arms are thrown forcibly backward, so that the backs of the hands may approach each other as nearly as possible. These motions, also, are to be repeatedly and rather quickly performed. Another extension motion, similarly added, consists in swinging the right arm in a circle, in which, beginning from the pendent position, the arm is carried upward in front, by the side of the head, and downward behind, the object being in the latter part of this course to throw it as directly backward as possible. The same is then done with the left arm. Lastly, both arms are thus exercised together. These motions are performed quickly.

———

THE INDIAN CLUB EXERCISES

THE PORTION ADOPTED
IN THE ARMY

One. A club is held by the handle, pendent on each side (Plate II. *fig.* 1); that in the right hand is carrried over the head and left shoulder, until it hangs perpendicularly on the right side of the spine (Plate II. *fig.* 2); that in the left hand is carried over the former, in exactly the opposite direction (Plate II. *fig.* 2), until it hangs on the opposite side; holding both clubs still pendent, the hands are raised somewhat higher than the head (Plate II. *fig.* 3); with the clubs in the same position, both arms are extended outward and backward (Plate II. *fig.* 6); they are lastly dropped into the first position. All this is done slowly.

Two. Commencing from the same position, the ends of both clubs are swung upward until they are held, vertically and side by side, at arm's length in front of the body, the hands being as high as the shoulders (Plate II. *fig.* 4); they are next carried in the same position, at arm's length, and on the same level, as far backward as possible (Plate II. *fig.* 5); each is then dropped backward until it hangs vertically downward (Plate II. *fig.* 6); and this exercise ends as the first. Previous, however, to dropping the clubs backward, it greatly improves this exercise, by a turn of the wrist upward and backward, to carry the clubs into a horizontal position behind the shoulders, so that, if long enough, their ends would touch (Plate III. *fig.* 1); next, by a turn of the wrist outward and downward, to carry them horizontally outward (Plate III. *fig.* 2); then by a turn of the wrist

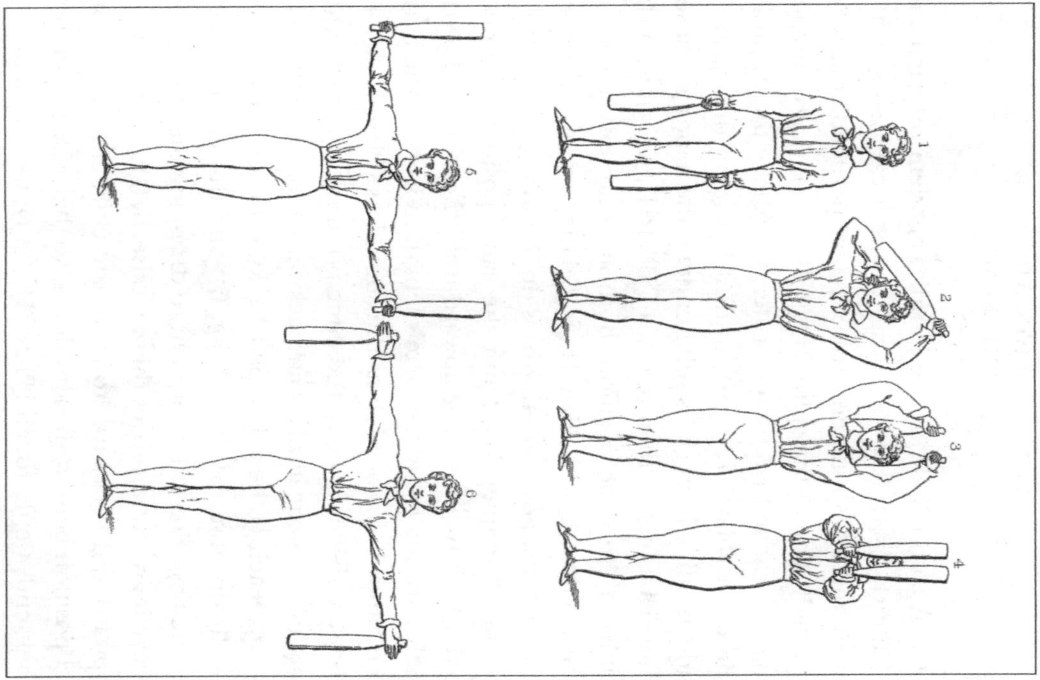

PLATE II

upward and forward, to carry them into a horizontal position before the breast (Plate III. *fig.* 3); again to carry them horizontally outward; and finally to drop them backward as already explained; and thence to the first position. All this is also done slowly.

Three. The clubs are to be swung by the sides, first separately, and then together, exactly as the hands were in the last extension motion.

THE NEW AND MORE BEAUTIFUL PORTION NOW ADDED FROM THE INDIAN PRACTICE

One. A club is held forward and upright in each hand, the forearm being placed horizontally, by the haunch on each side (Plate IV. *fig.* 1); both are thrown in a circle upward, forward, and, by a turn of the wrist, downward and backward, so as to strike under the arms (Plate IV. *fig.* 2); by an opposite movement, both are thrown back again in a similar circle, till they swing over the shoulders (Plate IV. *fig.* 3); and this movement is continued as long as agreeable.

Two. The clubs are held obliquely upward in each hand, lying on the front of the arms (Plate IV. *fig.* 4); that in the right hand is allowed to fall backward (Plate IV. *fig.* 5); and swings downward, forward to the extent of the arm, and as high as the head (Plate IV. *fig.* 6); the moment this club begins to return from this point, in precisely the same direction, to the front of the arm, that in the left hand is allowed to drop backward, and to perform the advancing portion of this course in the time that the other performs the returning portion, so that each is at the same time swinging in an opposite direction.

PLATE III

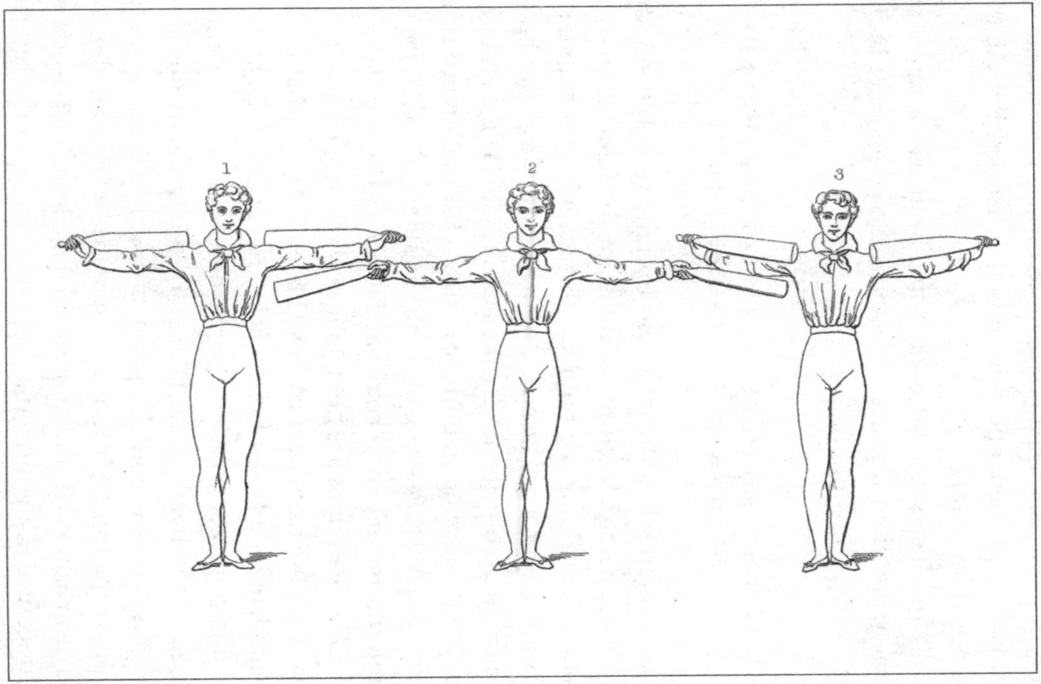

INDIAN CLUB EXERCISES

PLATE IV

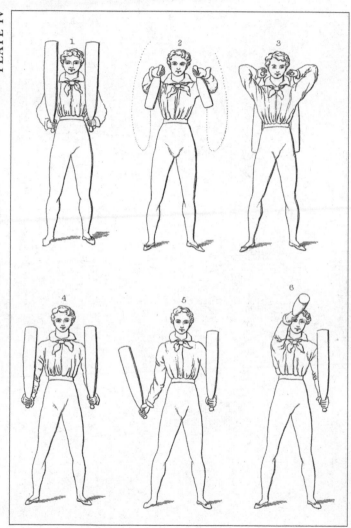

INDIAN CLUB EXERCISES

PLATE V

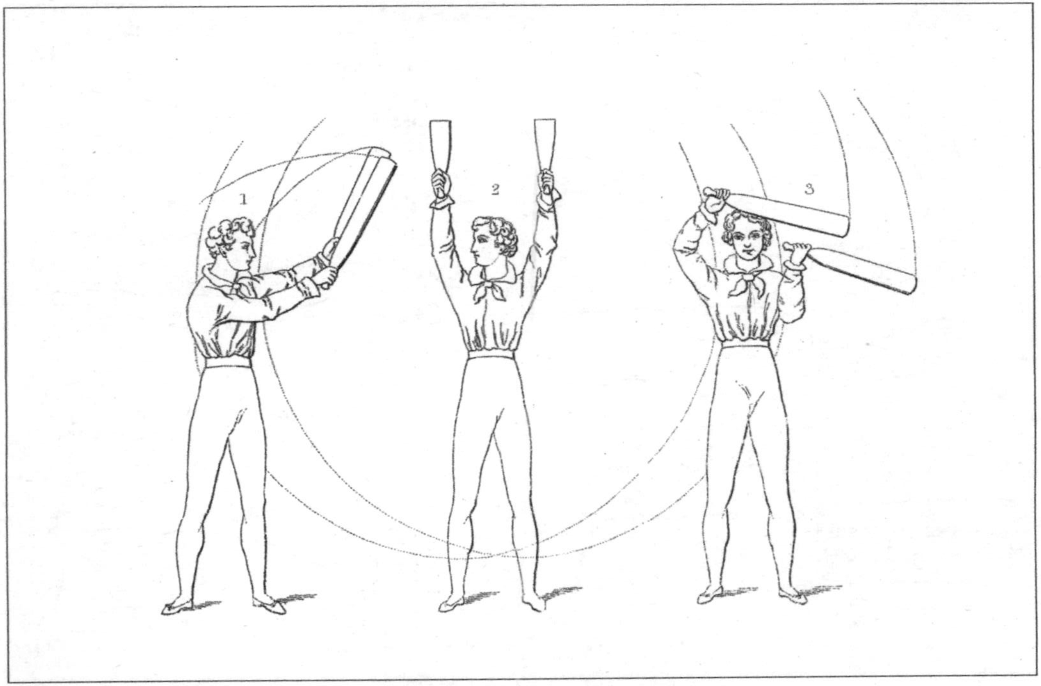

INDIAN CLUB EXERCISES

Three. From either of the first positions now given, the clubs are, by a turn of the body and extension of the arms, thrown upward and laterally (Plate V. *fig.* 1); make, at the extent of the arms, and in front of the figure, a circle in which they sweep downward by the feet and upward over the head (Plate V. *fig.* 2), and fall in a more limited curve towards the side on which they began (Plate V. *fig.* 3), in such a manner that the outer one forming a circle around the shoulder and the inner one round the head (both passing swiftly through the position in the last figure of the first exercise) they return to the first position; this is repeated to the other side; and so on alternately.

Four. Beginning from either first position, the body being turned laterally, for example, to the left, the club in the right hand is thrown upward in that direction at the full extent of the arm (Plate VI. *fig.* 1), and makes the large circle in front and curve behind as in the last exercise (Plate VI. *fig.* 2), while the club in the left hand makes at the same time a smaller circle in front of the head and behind the shoulders (Plate VI. *figs.* 1, 2, and 3), until crossing each other before the head (rather on the right side), their movements are exactly reversed, the club in the right hand performing the small circle round the head, while that in the left performs the large one, and these continue to be repeated to each side alternately.

Five. The clubs being in either first position, the body is turned to one side, the left, for example, and the clubs being thrown out in the same direction, make each, by a turn of the wrist, circle three times on the outer side of the outstretched arms (Plate VII. *fig.* 1); when completing the third circle, the clubs are thrown higher to the same

PLATE VI

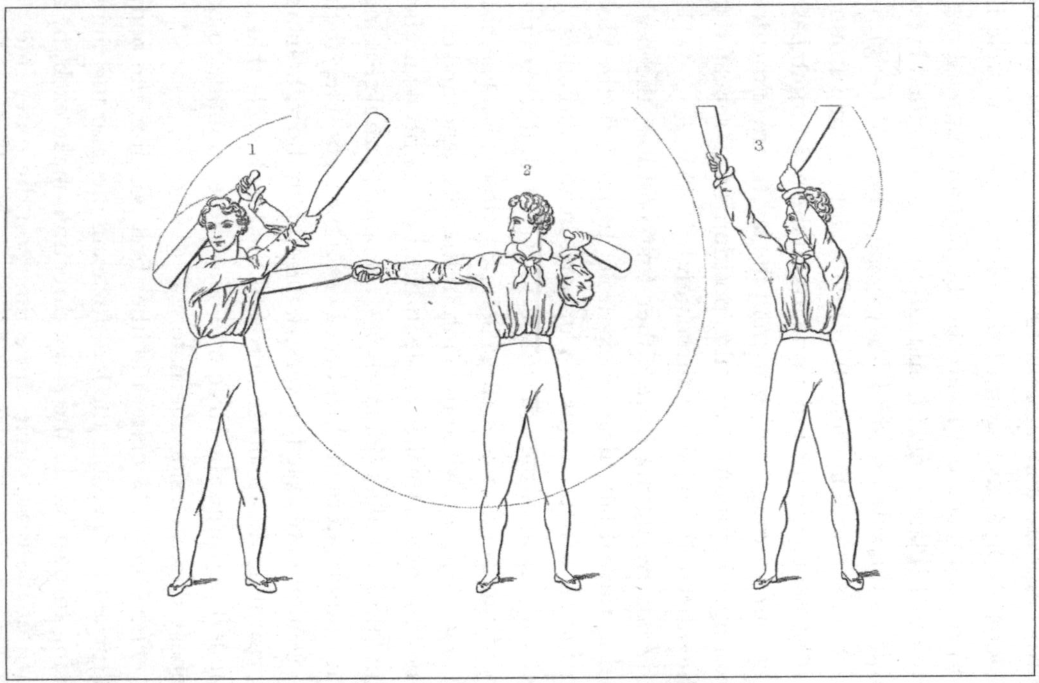

INDIAN CLUB EXERCISES

PLATE VII

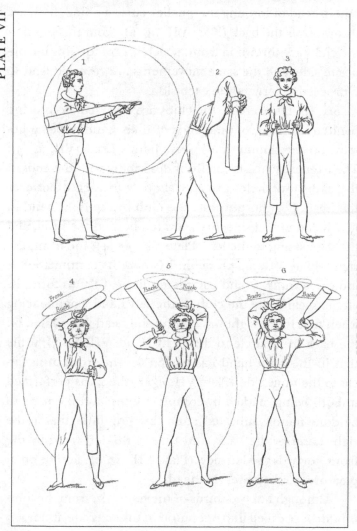

side, sweeping together in the large circle in front, as in the second exercise, the body similarly turning to the right; but, instead of forming the smaller curve behind, both are thrown over the back (Plate VII. *fig.* 2); from this position the clubs are thrown in front, which is now towards the opposite side, and the same movements are reversed; and so it proceeds alternately to each side.

Six. In this exercise, the clubs are reversed, both being pendent in front, but the ends of their handles being upward on the thumb sides of the hands (Plate VII. *fig.* 3). The exercise consists chiefly in describing with the ends of the clubs two circles placed obliquely to each other over the head. For this purpose, the club in the right hand is, in a sweep to that side, first elevated behind the head, and thence passing to the left (Plate VII. *fig.* 4); the front, the right (Plate VII. *fig.* 5), behind (where its continuation is indicated in *fig.* 5, and completed in *fig.* 6) thus forms its circle; meanwhile the club in the left hand, commencing when that in the right was behind the head, has passed on the back of its circle to the right (Plate VII. *fig.* 5); while that in the right hand has passed on the front of its circle to the same side (Plate VII. *fig.* 5, the parts performed in both being marked by complete lines, and the parts to be done merely indicated); and they continue, that in the right hand by the back, and that in the left hand by the front, towards the left side (Plate VII. *fig.* 6), and so on at pleasure, circling over the head.

[Although but two-thirds of the body, viz. from the loins upward, are called into operation in this exercise, its importance must be estimated by the fact that they are precisely those requiring constant artificial practice, being naturally most exempted from exertion. As an adjunct to TRAINING, there is nothing in the whole round of gymnastic performances that will be found of more essential service than this exercise with the Indian clubs. It demands but little muscular exertion, and such as it does require calls chiefly upon that portion of the system which it finds in a state of comparative repose.]

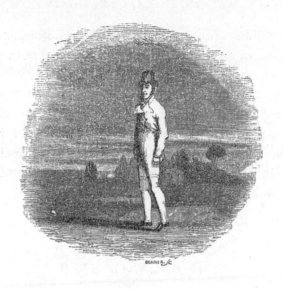

LOCOMOTIVE EXERCISES

In walking, the position is nearly the same as that already described under the POSITION heading.

The head should be upright, easy, and capable of free motion, right, left, up, or down, without affecting the body. The body must be kept erect and square to the front, having the breast projected, and the stomach retracted, though not so as to injure either freedom of respiration or ease of attitude. The shoulders should be kept moderately and equally back and low; and the arms should hang unconstrainedly by the sides. The balance on the limbs must be perfect. The knees straight, and the toes turned out as described, the weight of the body should be thrown forward,

as this facilitates progression. The military position in walking does not essentially differ from this, except in points
that exclusively regard the soldier; as that the head be kept
well up, and straight to the front, and the eyes not turned
to the right or left; the arms and hands kept perfectly steady
by the sides, and on no account suffered to move or vibrate:
care, however, being taken that the hand does not cling to
the thigh, or partake in the least degree of the movement
of the limb.

THE BALANCE STEP

THE object of this is to teach the free movement of the
limbs, preserving at the same time perfect squareness of
the shoulders, with the utmost steadiness of body; and no
labour is spared to attain this first and most essential object,
which forms, indeed, the very foundation of good walking.
The instructor must be careful that a habit be not contracted of drooping or throwing back a shoulder at these
motions, which are intended practically to show the true
principles of walking, and that steadiness of body is compat-
ible with perfect freedom in the limbs.

I. WITHOUT GAINING GROUND

To ensure precision, the military words of command are
prefixed.

Caution – Balance step without gaining ground, commencing with the left foot. The left foot is brought gently

forward with the toe at the proper angle to the left, the foot about three inches from the ground, the left heel in line with the toe of the right foot.

Rear – When steady, the left foot is brought gently back (without a jerk), the left knee a little bent, the left toe brought close to the right heel. The left foot in this position will not be so flat as to the front, as the toe will be a little depressed.

Front – When steady, the word Front will be given as above, and repeated to the rear three or four times.

Halt – To prevent fatigue, the word Halt will be given, when the left foot, either advanced, or to the rear, will be brought to the right. The instructor will afterwards cause the balance to be made on the left foot, advancing and retiring the right in the same manner.

2. GAINING GROUND BY THE WORD 'FORWARD'

Front – On the word Front, the left foot is brought gently to the front, without a jerk; the knee gradually straightened as the foot is brought forward, the toe turned out a little to the left, and remaining about three inches from the ground. This posture is continued for a few seconds only in the first instance, till practice gives steadiness in the position.

Forward – On this word of command, the left foot is brought to the ground, at about thirty inches from heel to heel, while the right foot is raised at the same moment, and continues extended to the rear. The body remains upright, but inclining forward; the head erect, and neither turned to the right nor left.

Front – On the word Front, the right foot is brought forward, and so on.

WALKING

OF all exercises, this is the most simple and easy. The weight of the body rests on one foot, while the other is advanced; it is then thrown upon the advanced foot, while the other is brought forward; and so on in succession. In this mode of progression, the slowness and equal distribution of motion is such, that many muscles are employed in a greater or lesser degree; each acts in unison with the rest; and the whole remains compact and united. Hence, the time of its movements may be quicker or slower, without deranging the union of the parts, or the equilibrium of the whole. It is owing to these circumstances, that walking displays so much of the character of the walker, that it is light and gay in women and children, steady and grave in men and elderly persons, irregular in the nervous and irritable, measured in the affected and formal, brisk in the sanguine, heavy in the phlegmatic, and proud or humble, bold or timid, &c., in strict correspondence with individual character.

The utility of walking exceeds that of all other modes of progression. While the able pedestrian is independent of stage coaches and hired horses, he alone fully enjoys the scenes through which he passes, and is free to dispose of his time as he pleases. To counterbalance these advantages, greater fatigue is doubtless attendant on walking: but this fatigue is really the result of previous inactivity; for daily exercise, gradually increased, by rendering walking more easy and agreeable, and inducing its more frequent practice, diminishes fatigue in such a degree, that very great distances may be accomplished with pleasure, instead of painful exertion.

Moderate walking exercises the most agreeable influence over all the functions. In relation to health, walking accelerates respiration and circulation, increases the temperature and cutaneous exhalation, and excites appetite and healthful nutrition. Hence, as an anonymous writer observes, the true pedestrian, after a walk of twenty miles, comes in to breakfast with freshness on his countenance, healthy blood coursing in every vein, and vigour in every limb, while the indolent and inactive man, having painfully crept over a mile or two, returns to a dinner which he cannot digest. In all individuals, walking is indispensably joined with the exercise of one or more of the external senses. It receives from the cerebral faculties a powerful influence, by which it is either accelerated or prolonged. Walking upon soft, even ground, at a moderate pace, is an exercise that may be taken without inconvenience, and even with advantage, after a meal. It is adapted for convalescents, who are not yet allowed to take stronger exercise. A firm, yet easy and graceful walk, is by no means common. There are few men who walk well if they have not learnt to regulate their motions by the lessons of a master, and this instruction is still more necessary for ladies. Having, now, therefore, taken a general view of the character and utility of walking, I subjoin some more particular remarks on the

GENERAL MECHANISM OF WALKING

For the purpose of walking, we first bear upon one leg the weight of the body, which pressed equally on both. The other leg is then raised, and the foot quits the ground by rising from the heel to the point. For that purpose, the leg must be bent upon the thigh, and the thigh upon the pelvis: the foot is then carried straight forward, at a sufficient height to clear the ground without grazing it. To render it possible, however, to move this foot, the haunch, which rested with its weight upon the thigh, must turn forward and out. As soon as, by this movement, this foot has passed the other, it must be extended on the leg, and the leg upon the thigh, and in this manner, by the lengthening of the whole member, and without being drawn back, it reaches the ground at a distance in advance of the other foot, which is more considerable according to the length of the step, and it is placed so softly on the ground as not to jerk or shake the body in the slightest degree. As soon as the foot which has been placed on the ground becomes firm, the weight of the body is transported to the limb on that side, and the other foot, by a similar mechanism, is brought forward in its turn. In all walking, the most important circumstance is that the body incline forward, and that the movement of the leg and thigh spring from the haunch, and be free and natural. Viewed in this way, the feet have been well compared to the spokes of a wheel: the weight of the body falling upon them alternately.

This exercise puts in action the extensors and flexors of the thighs and legs, a great number of the muscles of the

PLATE VIII

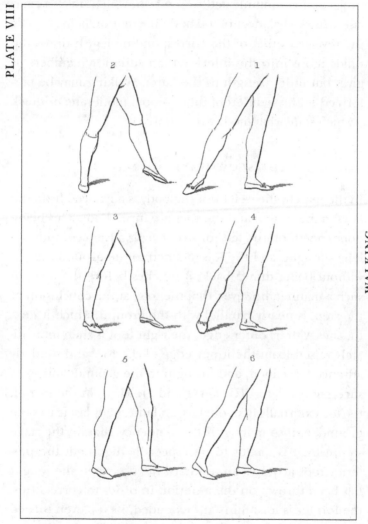

trunk, and more or less those of the shoulders, according to the rapidity of the pace, and the greater or lesser degree of projection communicated to the arm, which, in this exercise, acts as a balancer of the body, the motion being exactly the reverse of that of the corresponding leg. It draws the fluids more into the inferior than superior members: it gives but little strength to the latter. Walking may be performed in three different times – slow, moderate, or quick – which somewhat modify its action.

THE SLOW WALK, OR MARCH

In the march, the weight of the body is advanced from the heel to the instep, and the toes are turned out. This being done, one foot, the left for instance, is advanced, with the knee straight, and the toe inclined to the ground, which, without being drawn back, it touches before the heel, in such a manner, however, that the sole, at the conclusion of the step, is nearly parallel with the ground, which it next touches with its outer edge; the right foot is then immediately raised from the inner edge of the toe, and similarly advanced, inclined, and brought to the ground; and so in succession (Plate VIII. *figs*. 1 and 2). Thus, in the march, the toe externally first touches, and internally last leaves the ground; and so marked is this tendency, that, in the stage step, which is meant to be especially dignified, the posterior foot acquires an awkward flexure when the weight has been thrown on the anterior. In order to correct this, the former is for an instant extended, its toe even turned backward and outward, and its tip internally alone rested on the ground, previous to its being in its turn advanced.

Thus the toe's first touching and last leaving the ground is peculiarly marked in this grandest form of the march. This pace should be practised until it can be firmly and gracefully performed.

THE MODERATE AND THE QUICK PACE

These will be best understood by a reference to the pace which we have just described; the principal difference between them being as to the advance of the weight of the body, the turning out of the toes, and the part of the foot which first touches and last leaves the ground. We shall find that the times of these two paces require a further advance of the weight, and suffer successively less and less of turning out the toes, and of this extended touching with the toe, and covering the ground with the foot.

THE MODERATE PACE

Here the weight of the body is advanced from the heel to the ball of the foot; the toes are less turned out; and it is no longer the toe, but the ball of the foot, which first touches and last leaves the ground; its outer edge, or the ball of the little toe, first breaking the descent of the foot, and its inner edge, or the ball of the great toe, last projecting the weight (Plate VIII. *figs.* 3 and 4). Thus, in this step, less of the foot may be said actively to cover the ground; and this adoption of nearer and stronger points of support and action is essential to the increased quickness and exertion of the pace.

The mechanism of this pace has not been sufficiently attended to. People pass from the march to the quick pace they know not how; and hence all the awkwardness and embarrassment of their walk when their pace becomes moderate, and the misery they endure when this pace has to be performed by them, unaccompanied, up the middle of a long and well-lighted room, where the eyes of a brilliant assembly are exclusively directed to them. Let those who have felt this but attend to what we have here said: the motion of the arms and of every other part depends on it.

THE QUICK PACE

Here, the weight of the body is advanced from the heel to the toes; the toes are least turned out; and still nearer and stronger points of support and action are chosen. The outer edge of the heel first touches the ground, and the sole of the foot projects the weight.

These are essential to the increased quickness of this pace (Plate VIII. *figs.* 5 and 6); and it is important to remark, as to all these paces, that the weight is successively more thrown forward, and the toes are successively less turned out. In the grandest form of the march, the toes, as we have seen, are, in the posterior foot, though but for a moment, even thrown backward; in the moderate pace, they have an intermediate direction; and in the quick pace, they are thrown more directly forward, as in the six figures of Plate VIII.

It is this direction of the toes, and still more the nearer and stronger points of support and action, namely, the heel and sole of the foot, which are essential to the quick pace so universally practised, but which, together with the great inclination of the body, being ridiculously transferred to the moderate pace, make unfortunate people look so awkward, as we shall now explain. The time of the moderate pace is, as it were, filled up by the more complicated process of the step – by the gradual and easy breaking of the descent of the foot on its outer edge, or the ball of the little toe, by the deliberate positing of the foot, by its equally gradual and easy projection from its inner edge, or the ball of the great toe. The quick pace, if its time be lengthened, has no such filling up: the man stumps at once down on his heel, and could rise instantly from his sole, but finds that, to fill up his time, he must pause an instant; he feels he should do something, and does not know what; his hands suffer the same momentary paralysis as his feet; he gradually becomes confused and embarrassed: deeply sensible of this, he at last exhibits it externally; a smile or a titter arises, though people do not well know at what; but, in short, the man has walked like a clown, because the mechanism of his step has not filled up its time, or answered its purpose.

I trust that the mechanism and time of the three paces are here simply, clearly, and impressively described. The following is the more imperfect, but still useful, military description, with its words of command.

SLOW STEP

March. On the word March, the left foot is carried thirty inches to the front, and, without being drawn back, is placed softly on the ground, so as not to jerk or shake the body; seventy-five of these steps to be taken in a minute.

(The recruit is ordered to be carefully trained, and thoroughly instructed in this step, as an essential foundation for arriving at accuracy in the paces of more celerity. This is the slowest step at which troops are to move.)

QUICK STEP

The cadence of the slow pace having become perfectly habitual, a quick time is next taught, which is 108 steps in a minute, each of thirty inches, making 270 feet in a minute.

Quick March. The command Quick March being given with a pause between them, the word Quick is to be considered as a caution, and the whole to remain perfectly steady. On the word March, the whole move off, conforming to the directions already given. (This pace is applied generally to all movements by large as well as small bodies of troops; and therefore the recruit is trained and thoroughly instructed in this essential part of his duty.)

DOUBLE MARCH

The directions for the march apply, in a great degree, to this step, which is 150 steps in a minute, each of thirty-six inches, making 450 feet in a minute.

Double March. On the words Double March, the whole step off together with the left feet, keeping the head erect, and the shoulders square to the front; the knees are a little bent; the body is more advanced than in the other marches; the arms hang with ease down the outside of the thighs. The person marching is carefully habituated to the full pace of thirty-six inches, otherwise he gets into the habit of a short trot, which defeats the obvious advantages of this degree of march. In the army, great advantage attends the constant use of the plummet; and the several lengths swinging the times of the different marches in a minute, are as follows:

				In Hun
Slow time	·	·	75 steps in the minute	24,96
Quick time	·	·	108 " "	12,03
Double march	·	150 " "		6,26

A musket ball, suspended by a string which if not subject to stretch, and on which are marked the different required lengths, answers the above purpose, may be easily acquired, and is directed to be frequently compared with an accurate standard in the adjutant's possession. The length of the plummet is to be measured from the point of suspension to the centre of the ball. In practising all these paces, the pupils should also be accustomed to march upon a narrow plane, where there is room for only one foot, upon rough, uneven ground, and on soft ground which yields to the foot.

Walking exercises a greater influence over the economy when it takes place on inclined planes than on a flat surface. In ascending, the effort is made in a direction directly opposed to the general tendency of heavy bodies: the body is strongly bent, the upper part of the trunk in advance; the action of the posterior and anterior muscles of the thigh is considerable; and circulation and respiration are speedily accelerated by the violence of the muscular contractions. In descending, on the contrary, effort is requisite to keep up the body, which tends to obey the laws of gravitation; and to moderate the tendency of gravity to project forward in the centre, the body is thrown back, the sacrospinal mass, and the posterior muscles of the neck, are strongly contracted, the knees bent, and the steps much shorter. Men with long, flat feet, and the heel bone little projecting, are bad walkers.

FEATS IN WALKING

The power of walking great distances without fatigue is an important matter, in which the English have of late excelled. A good walker will do six miles an hour, for one hour, on a good road.[1] If in perfect training, he may even do twelve miles in two hours. Eighteen miles in three hours is a much more doubtful affair, though some are said to have achieved it.

A Cork paper, of recent date, describes a match of ten miles in 120 minutes, on the Mallow and Fermoy Road, by Captain John T. G. Campbell, of the 91st (Argyleshire) Regiment, accoutred in heavy marching order of a private soldier, viz. with knapsack and kit, great-coat and mess-tin, musket, bayonet, and sixty rounds of ball cartridge: total, fifty pounds' weight. Heavy bets were pending on the issue. The captain started at eight o'clock, a. m., and performed this undertaking in the short time of 107 minutes and a quarter, thus winning the match, and having twelve minutes and three quarters to spare.

At the rate of five miles an hour, pedestrians of the first class will do forty miles in eight hours, and perhaps fifty in ten.[2]

1. Seven miles in one hour are said to have been done by some.

2. A clever writer in Blackwood's Magazine says, 'There can be no doubt that, out of the British army, on a war establishment, ten thousand men might be chosen, by trial, who would compose a corps

At the rate of four miles an hour, a man may walk any length of time. Robert Skipper walked 1,000 miles in 1,000 successive half-hours; on the same ground Captain Barclay walked 1,000 miles in 1,000 successive hours.

In the art of walking quickly, the circumstance perhaps most important is, to keep the knees somewhat bent and springy.

————————

RUNNING

'RUNNING,' says one of our gymnasiarchs, 'only differs from walking by the rapidity of the movement.' This is quite incorrect. Running is precisely intermediate to walking and leaping; and, in order to pass into it from walking, the motion must be changed. A series of leaps from each foot alternately must be performed, in order to constitute it; the foot which is left behind quits the ground before the foot in advance is firmly fixed, so that the centre of gravity remains uncertain in passing from one leg to the other, which forms a series of leaps, and renders a fall a common occurrence.

————————

capable of marching fifty miles a day, on actual service, for a whole week. The power of such a corps is not to be calculated: it would far outgo cavalry.'

PLATE IX

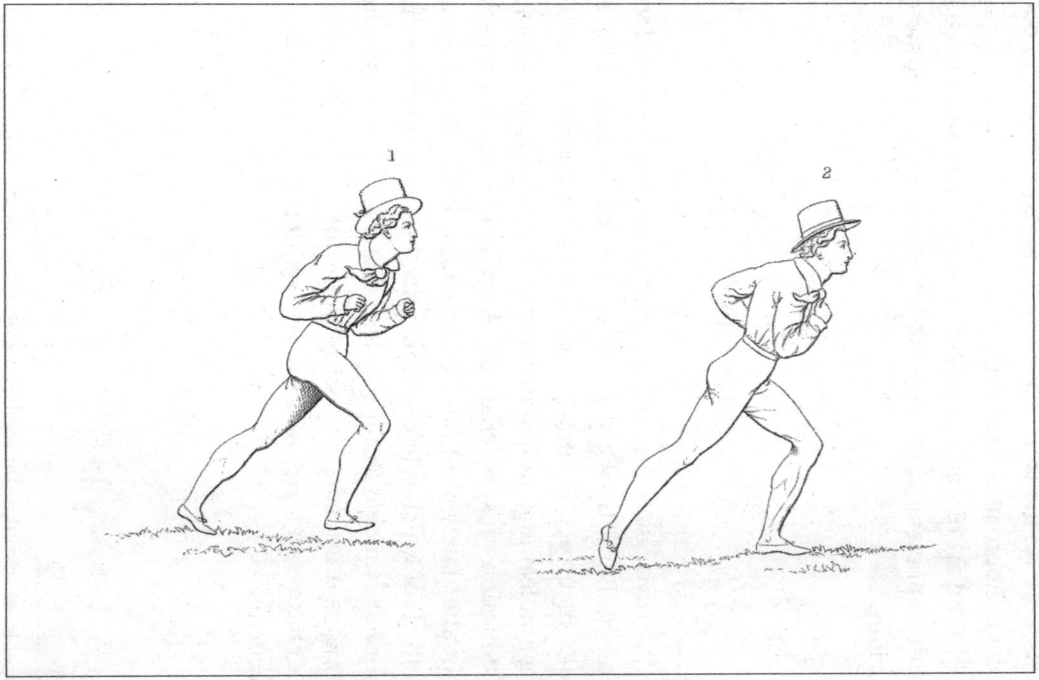

RUNNING

POSITION IN RUNNING

The upper part of the body is slightly inclined forward; the head slightly thrown backward, to counteract the gravity forward: the breast is freely projected; the shoulders are steady, to give a fixed point to the auxiliary muscles of respiration: the upper parts of the arm are kept near the sides; the elbows are bent, and each forms an acute angle; the hands are shut, with the nails turned inward; and the whole arms move but slightly, in order that the muscles of respiration on the chest may be as little as possible disturbed, and follow only the impulse communicated by other parts (Plate IX. *fig.* 1). There exists, in fact, during the whole time of running, a strong and permanent contraction of the muscles of the shoulder and arm, which, though very violent, is less serviceable to the extended movements, than to keep the chest immoveable, towards which the arms are brought close, the flexors and adductors of which are especially contracted.

ACTION IN RUNNING

At every step, the knees are stretched out; the legs kept as straight as possible; the feet almost graze the ground; the tread is neither with the mere balls of the toes, nor with the whole sole of the foot; and the spring is made rapidly from one foot to the other, so that they pass each other with great velocity (Plate IX. *fig.* 2).

But the abdominal members are not the only ones in motion, although it is in them that the greatest development

takes place. Throughout the whole time of running, a strong
and permanent contraction of the muscles of the shoulder,
arm, and forearm takes place; this, though very violent, is
less for the purpose of aiding motion than of preserving the
immobility of the thorax, which is pressed upon the whole
thoracic member, whose flexors and adductors are strongly
contracted. The degree of velocity, however, must be proportioned to the length of the steps. Too slow and long, as
well as too quick and short, steps, may be equally injurious.

RESPIRATION

Speed, and still more duration in running, are in proportion to the development of the lungs, and consequently the
volume of oxygen and blood which they can combine in
their parenchyma at each respiratory movement. Thus, of
two men, one having the abdominal members developed,
and the other possessing good lungs, the former will run
with the greatest speed for a short distance, but if the distance be considerable, he will soon be gained upon by the
latter. A runner, after performing a certain space, is seized
with a difficulty of breathing, long before the repetition
of the contractions has produced fatigue in the abdominal
members. To excel, therefore, in running, requires, like
walking and dancing, a peculiar exercise. As the muscular
contractions depend, for their principle of excitement, on
the respiration, the chest should be firmly fixed, so as both
to facilitate this, and to serve as a point of support for the
efforts of the lower members. The best runners are those
who have the *best wind*, and keep the breast dilated for the
longest time.

During the whole time of running, long inspirations and slow expirations are of the greatest importance; and young persons cannot be too early accustomed to them. To facilitate respiration towards the end of the race, the upper part of the body may be leant a little forward, Running should cease as soon as the breath becomes very short, and a strong perspiration takes place.

MODERATE RUNNING

This is performed gently and in equal time, and may be extended to a considerable space. In practising this pace, it is necessary to fix the distance to be run; and this should always be proportioned to the age and strength of the runners. This exercise, more than all others, requires to be proceeded with in a progressive manner. If, at the first trial, you run too fast or too long a time, it may produce spitting of blood and headache, or aneurysms of the heart and principal vessels, especially if the weather be dry and cold.

A moderately cool day may accordingly be chosen, a distance of three hundred feet measured, and the runners placed in a line at one end. They may then start, trot at the rate of about seven feet in a second to the opposite end, turn, and continue until they reach the spot whence they started. Frequent repetition of this is sufficient at first. Afterwards, they may run over this space, two, three, or four times without stopping; and the exercise may then be limited to this. It may, on subsequent days, be extended to five, six, and seven times the distance.

Fatigue is then generally quite removed; and the run may either be continued farther, or the runners, if neither heated nor winded, may accelerate their pace. They may next attempt a mile in ten minutes; and repeat this, till, being gradually less and less heated, they can either extend the distance, or diminish the time, in any measured proportion. At this pace, six miles may afterwards be run in an hour.

RAPID RUNNING

This is best applied to a short space in a little time. Three hundred feet upon an open plain will not generally be found too great. At each end of this, a cross line may be drawn, and the runners may arrange themselves on one line, while the umpire is placed at the other. On the latter giving the signal, the running commences, and he who first passes him gains the race. It is extremely useful always to run beyond the line at a gentler pace, as it gradually lowers the actions of the respiratory and circulating systems.

Running is more easy on a level surface, but should be practised on ground of every variety: upon long, square, and circular plots of ground. The pupils should be accustomed to turn promptly out of the direct line – a faculty not possessed by animals, and exceedingly useful when pursued. They should also run up hill, and particularly down, as it is dangerous unless frequently practised.

FEATS IN RUNNING

The practice of running may be carried to a great degree of perfection.

A quarter of a mile in a minute is good running; and a mile in four minutes, at four starts, is excellent.

The mile was perhaps never run in four minutes, but it has been done in four minutes and a half.[3]

A mile in five minutes is good running. Two miles in ten minutes is oftener failed in than accomplished. Four miles in twenty is said to puzzle the cleverest.

Ten miles an hour is done by all the best runners. Fifteen miles in an hour and a half has never perhaps been done.

It is reported that West ran forty miles in five hours and a half. This, it is said, was done by one individual in four hours and three quarters, or less.

As to great distances, Rainer failed in two attempts to accomplish 100 miles in eighteen hours. West is said to have accomplished this.

EFFECTS OF RUNNING

In running, the mass of our organs is agitated by violent and constant shocks, which succeed with rapidity; but the abdominal members are not the only ones in motion, although they are those in which the development is most considerable. Running develops not only the abdominal members, but has a strong influence upon the respiratory parts. This exercise is particularly suited to young persons,

---

3. Half a mile was recently run in two minutes; but it was down a fall as precipitous as a mountain's side, and the performer was blind in the last twenty yards. – ED. Fifth Edition.

especially those of a lymphatic temperament. It should not, however, be practised after meals.

LEAPING

LEAPING consists principally in the sudden straightening of the articulations, performed by a strong and instantaneous contraction of the extensors, by which the body is rapidly projected from the ground.

The leaping-stand consists of two moveable posts, above six feet high, having, above the second foot from the ground, holes bored through them, at the distance of an inch from each other; two iron pins to be placed in the holes at any height; a cord, at least ten feet long, passed over these pins, and kept straight by two sand-bags at its ends; and weights upon the feet of the posts, to prevent them from falling (Plate X. *fig.* 1). The leap over the cord is made from the side of the stand towards which the heads of the pegs are turned; so that, if the feet touch the cord, it will easily and instantly fall.

In all kinds of leaping, it is of great importance to draw in and retain the breath at the moment of the greatest effort, as it gives the chest more solidity to support the rest of the members, impels the blood into the muscular parts, and increases their strength. The hands, also, should be shut, and the arms pendent. The extent of the leap in height, or horizontally, is proportioned to the power employed, and the practice acquired. As it is performed with facility only in proportion to the strength exerted, and the

PLATE X

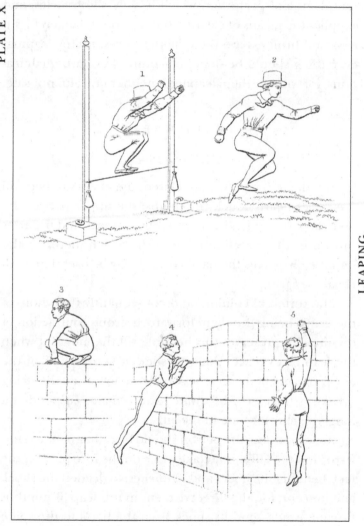

elasticity and suppleness of the articulations and muscles of the lower extremities, much exercise is necessary to attain that degree of perfection which lessens all obstacles, and supplies the means of clearing them without danger. Lightness and firmness are the qualities necessary for leaping: everything should be done to acquire these two qualifications, for without them leaping is neither graceful nor safe.

THE HIGH LEAP

Without a Run

In this, the legs and feet are closed; the knees are bent till the calves nearly touch the thighs; the upper part of the body, kept straight, is inclined a little forward; and the arms thrown in the direction of the leap, which increases the impulse, preserves the balance, and may be useful in a fall (Plate X. *fig.* 1).

The vertebral column, and consequently the whole of the trunk, being thus bent forward, a strong contraction of the muscles preserves this bending till the moment when the leap takes place; then, by sudden contraction of the extensors, the body stretches out like a bow when the string breaks, is thus jerked forward, and remains suspended a longer or shorter time in the air.

In descending, the person should be rather inclined forward; and the fall should take place on the fore part vof the feet, bending the knees and haunches, to deaden the shock and descent; for, the direct descent in this leap, if not thus broken, would send its shock from the heels to the spine and head, and might occasion injury. To perpendicularity in this leap, should be added lightness, so that scarcely any noise from the leap should be heard.

This leap, without a run, may be practised at the height:

1. Of the knees.
2. Of the middle of the thighs.
3. Of the hips.
4. Of the lower ribs.

With a Run

The run preceding the leap should never exceed ten paces, the distance between the point of springing and the cord being equal to half the cord's height from the ground. The view of the leaper should be directed first to the spot whence he is to spring; and, the moment he has reached that, to the cord, accustoming himself to spring from either foot, and from both feet.

The instant the spring is made, or (if it be made with one foot) immediately after, the feet should be closed, and the knees drawn forcibly towards the chin. Throughout, flexibility and skill, not violent exertion, should be displayed. This leap, with a run, may be practised at the height:

1. Of the hips.
2. Of the lower ribs.
3. Of the pit of the stomach.
4. Of the breast.
5. Of the chin.
6. Of the eyes.
7. Of the crown of the head.

Feats in High Leaping

A good high leaper will clear five feet; a first-rate one, five and a half; and an extraordinary one, six feet. Ireland is mentioned as having cleared an extended cord at the height of fourteen feet. Another man, it is said, jumped to the height of seventeen feet, which was three times the height of his own body.[4]

THE LONG LEAP

Without a Run

This is generally performed upon straight firm ground, on which there are marks, or parallel lines, at equal distances. The first of these lines is the place to leap from. The leapers succeed each other, and clear a greater number of lines, according to their strength and skill. Here the feet are closed; the whole weight rests upon the balls of the toes; and the body is inclined forward. Both arms are then swung forward, backward, then drawn strongly forward, and at the same instant the limbs, having been bent, are extended with the utmost possible force.

In performing this leap, the hands and body must be bent forward, especially at the end of the movement, when the leaper alights. On level ground, twelve feet is a good standing leap; and fourteen is one of comparatively rare occurrence.

4. The author means, with the aid of a spring-board. – ED. Fifth Edition.

With a Run

This leap is best executed with a run; and we have therefore dwelt less upon the former. Here, also, the body must be inclined forward.

The run should be made over a piece of firm, and not slippery ground, to the extent of ten, fifteen, or twenty paces; should consist of small steps, increasing in quickness as they approach the point of springing; and these should be so calculated as to bring upon the point that foot with which the leaper is accustomed to spring. The spring, as here implied, should be performed with one foot, and the arms thrown forcibly towards the place proposed to be reached. The height, as well as the length of the leap, must be calculated; for the leap is shortened by not springing a proper height (Plate X. *fig.* 2).

In the descent, the feet are closed, the knees bent, the upper part of the body inclined forward, and the toes first touch the ground, at which moment, a light spring, and afterwards some short steps, are made, in order to avoid any sudden check. In a much extended leap, however, alighting on the toes is impossible. A sort of horizontal swing is then achieved, by which the leaper's head is little higher than his feet, and his whole figure is almost parallel with the ground; and, in this case, to alight on the toes is impossible. Care must here be taken not to throw the feet so much forward as to cause the leaper to fall backward at the moment of descent. The ground must be cleared, or the leap is imperfect and unfair.

This leap may be practised at:

1. Double the length of the body.
2. Twice and a half that length.
3. Three times that length.

Feats in Long Leaping

On level ground, twenty feet is a first-rate leap; twenty-one is extraordinary; and twenty-two is very rarely accomplished.[5] With a run and a leap, on a slightly inclined plane, twenty-three feet have been done.

Of the various kinds of leaps, the first or simple leap, which is produced principally by the extension of the abdominal members (which impel the body either straight upward, in the vertical leap, or obliquely upward and forward, in the horizontal or rather parabolic leap) requires, in addition to the contraction of the abdominal members (especially if the leap be executed with the feet close together) a violent action of the muscles of the abdomen, upper parts of the back, anterior parts of the loins, and of the thorax and shoulders.

THE DEEP LEAP

This may be made either with or without the hands. In either way, to avoid the shock, the body must be kept in a bent position, and the fall be upon the balls of the toes. When the hands are used, the leaper places them in front

5. I have seen twenty-two feet covered forward and backward, by an Irish tailor. – ED. Fifth Edition.

of the feet; and during the descent, the weight of the body
is checked by the former, and passes in a diminished state
to the latter; so that the shock is obviated.

A flight of steps serves the purpose of this exercise.
The leaper ascends a certain number; leaps from the side;
gradually increases the number; and, by practising progres-
sively higher, finds it easy to leap from heights which at first
appalled him. He afterwards combines the long and deep
leaps. For this purpose, a rivulet, which has one bank high
and the opposite one low, is very favourable. Children can
easily take a leap of nine feet in descending.

THE DEEP LEAP BACKWARD,
FROM A REST ON THE HANDS

This exercise is first performed from platforms of various
heights, and from walls of various elevations. The object is
to lessen the shock that the legs and body experience in
reaching the ground at a depth of more than six or seven
feet, and to diminish the distance, if possible, at the same
time that it diminishes the violence and velocity of the fall.
All this is easily managed by observing the following rules.

Suppose the pupil placed upon a platform of four or six
feet in height; he must first examine the place he is about
to leap to, so as to select the most favourable part, free from
stones and other obstacles. He will then approach the extremity of the platform, with his back towards it, and bend
his body, placing his hands in the position shown in Plate X.
fig. 3. Having taken up this position securely, he will lean
his head a little forward, raise his toes from the platform,
and remain for an instant supported by the arms. The body

then begins to extend, and the legs to lengthen downward and backward; the arms follow this movement, bend, and support the body by the hands, which have a secure resting-place on the edge of the platform, as in Plate X. *fig.* 4. This descending movement is executed as slowly as possible: the arms stretch out to their utmost length, till the body is sustained by the last phalanx of the fingers or touches the ground with the feet. If it does not reach the ground, the pupil drops gently down on the tips of his toes, bends himself, and recovers his upright position.

There is another mode of descending, when the last resting-place for the hands is the top of a counterfort, or prop on a wall without a counterfort. This consists (see Plate X. *fig.* 5) in seizing the last hold with the right hand, for instance, and in hanging firmly by that hand, whilst the left, being at liberty, is lowered and pushes back the body from the projecting stones in the walls, to prevent injury in the descent. The impulse thus given is, however, very trifling, and solely to avoid hurt, without increasing the violence of the fall, which ought to be facilitated on reaching the ground by the rules already given. By these means, the height of a wall is relatively diminished, for a man who hangs suspended by his arms, has six feet less to drop than he who has his feet where he might put his hands.

The down leap, unless gradually practised, may produce rupture of the diaphragm. When, however, the elevation from which the leap is taken is gradually increased, the eye becomes accustomed to measure the most extensive distances fearlessly. At the same time, by practice, the abdominal members learn to bend properly under the weight of the trunk, and thereby preserve the organs contained in it from serious injuries. In this kind of leap, the shocks will be diminished by retaining the air in the chest, which may be done by closing the glottis.

Persons who have long toes, powerful calves, and prominent heels, are the best adapted for leaping.

VAULTING

In vaulting, by a spring of the feet, the body is raised, and by leaning the hands upon a fixed object, it at the same time receives, in oblique vaulting, a swing which facilitates the action. As the inclination thus given to the body depends not merely on the feet, but on the hands, we have the power to guide the body in any direction.

This exercise is conveniently practised on the vaulting bar, which rests upon two or three posts. It may be performed with or without running. The beginner may at first be allowed a run of a few paces, ending in a preparatory spring; and he may afterwards be allowed only a spring.

OBLIQUE VAULTING

To mount, the vaulter must place himself in front of the bar; make a preparatory spring with the feet close; fix at that moment both hands upon the bar; heave himself up, and swing the right leg over. The body, supported by the hands, may then easily descend into the riding position. To dismount, the vaulter, supported by the hands, must extend the feet, make a little swing forward, and a greater one

PLATE XI

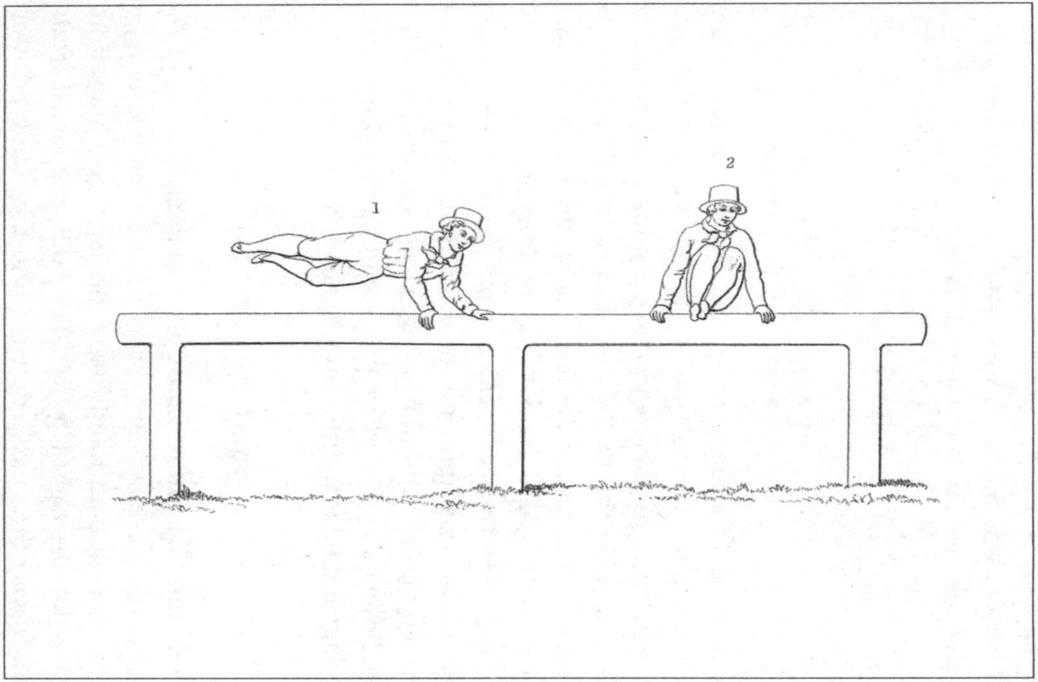

VAULTING

backward, so as to heave both feet behind over the bar, and spring to the ground with them close.

To do this, he must first clearly define to himself the place where he intends to fall. Then, having placed both hands upon the bar, he should first bend and then extend the joints, so as to raise the body with all his strength, and throw his legs, kept close, high over the bar (Plate XI. *fig.* 1). When the right hand (if he vault to the right) quits the bar, the left remains, the feet reach the ground on the opposite side, and he falls on both feet, with the knees projected, and the hands ready, if necessary, to break the fall.

In vaulting to the right, the left foot passes in the space which was between both hands, the right hand quits the bar, and the left guides the body in the descent. In vaulting to the left, the right foot passes in the space which was between both hands, the left hand quits the bar, and the right guides the body in its descent. As, however, it is difficult for beginners to vault either way, this is not to be attempted until after sufficient practice in the way which may be easiest. The vaulter may then, with a preparatory spring, try the following heights:

1. That of the pit of the stomach.
2. That of a middling-sized horse.
3. His own height or more.

STRAIGHT-FORWARD VAULTING

For this purpose, both hands must be placed at such distance on the bar as to give room for the feet between them; the body should be forcibly raised; the knees drawn up towards the breast; and the feet brought between the hands, without moving them from their place (Plate XI. *fig.* 2). This should be practised until it can be done easily.

This straight-forward vault may have three different terminations. When the feet are in the space between the hands, the vaulter may stand upright. He may pass his feet to the opposite side, whilst he seats himself. He may continue to leap over the seat, through the arms, letting both hands go at once after the legs have passed.

LEAPING WITH A POLE

THIS is a union of leaping and vaulting, in which the vaulter, instead of supporting himself upon a fixed object, carries with him a pole, which he applies to whatever spot he chooses. In supporting the body by a pole during the leap, a great deal also depends upon balancing, as well as on the strength of the arms and legs.

THE HIGH LEAP WITH A POLE

The pole prescribed for this exercise is the planed stem of a straight-grown fir, from seven to ten feet long, and about two inches thick at the bottom. Such a pole naturally diminishes towards the top; and it is better to plane off the lower end a little. Care must be taken that it be sufficiently strong; such as make a crackling noise during the leap should be immediately thrown aside.

PLATE XII

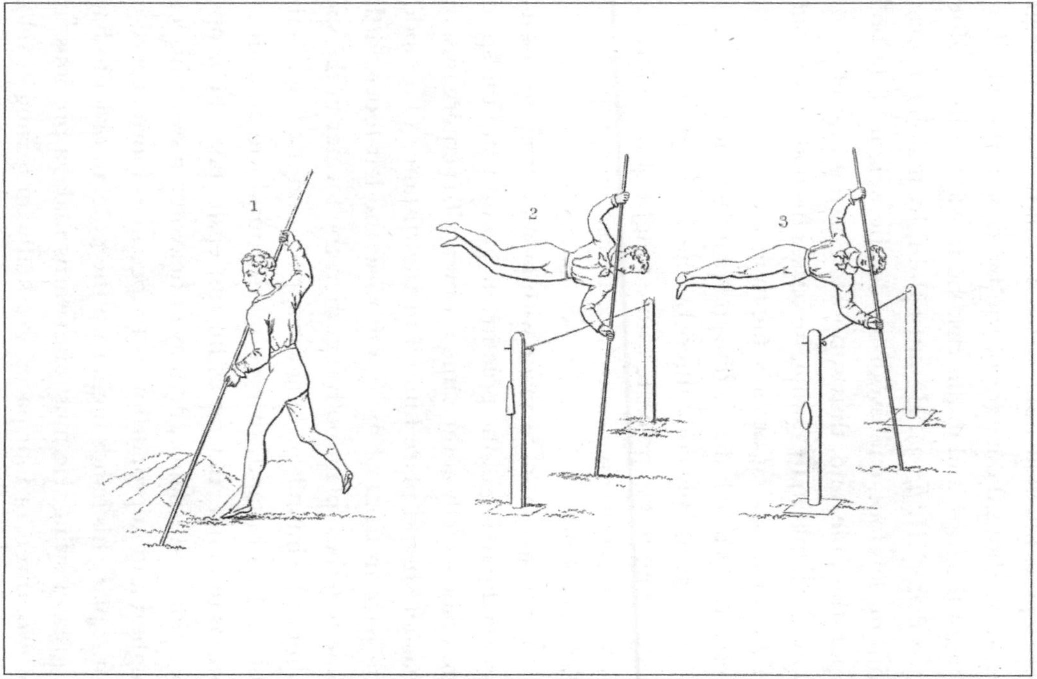

The learner, supposed to be already expert in leaping and vaulting, may at first place himself before a small ditch, with a pole, which he holds in such a manner, that the right hand be about the height of the head, and the left about that of the hips, and in this case he must fix it in the ditch (see Plate XII. *fig.* 1). He must then, by making a spring with his left foot, endeavour to rest the weight of his body upon the pole, and, thus supported, swing himself to the opposite bank. In this swing, he passes his body by the right of the pole, making, at the same time, a turn, so that, at the descent, his face is directed to the place whence he leaped. The faults usually committed by the beginner, consist in his trusting to the pole the whole weight of the body; and in losing the necessary purchase by keeping at too great a distance from it.

This leap cannot be made with proper force and facility unless the fixing of the pole in the ground and the spring are made exactly at the same moment. To acquire this, the learner should place himself at the distance of a moderate pace in front of the ditch; raise the left foot and the pole together; plant both together, the former in the spot whence he intends making the spring, and the latter in the ditch; then instantly swing himself round the pole, to the opposite bank. As soon as he can easily take the proper position and balance, he may endeavour to swing his legs higher; and in proportion as he becomes more expert, he must place his hands higher up the pole, in order to have a greater swing. He must afterwards make a previous run of two, three, or four paces, gradually increasing in velocity; and always taking care that the springing foot and the pole come to the ground at the same moment. When this difficulty is overcome, he may practise the exercise over the leaping-stand.

In leaping over the cord, the learner must take the pole in both hands; make a rather quick turn: conclude this with the spring, and planting the pole at the same moment; raise rapidly his whole body, by means of this spring and a powerful support on the pole, and swing over the cord; turning his body so that, at the descent, his face is directed to the place whence he sprung. This is a general description of the high leap; but it is necessary to explain the parts into which it may be divided, as follows:

One. In the handling the pole (Plate XII. *fig*. 1), it is immaterial, as to the lower hand, whether the thumb or the little finger be uppermost: the upper hand must have the thumb upward. The position of the upper hand is regulated by that of the lower one: as this advances higher up, the former must be proportionally raised. The lower hand then must be placed at a height proportionate to that of the leap: thus, if the latter be six feet, the lower hand must be at least from five and a half to six feet from the lower end of the pole. The leaper is, after a little practice, enabled to seize the pole in the proper way, from a mere glance at the leap.

Two. The preparatory run of from twelve to fifteen paces is accelerated as the leaper approaches the cord. Upon this run principally depend the facility and the success of the leap. As the spring can take place only with one foot, and as this must arrive correctly at the springing place, it is necessary that the order of the steps should be arranged so as to effect this object. If the leaper should be obliged to correct himself by making a few steps, either longer or shorter, just before making the spring, the leap is rendered difficult.

Three. The fixing of the pole in the ground, and the spring, must take place at the same instant, because by that means the upper and lower members operate together, no power is lost, and the swing is performed with the greatest facility. The place of the pole, however, varies with the height of the leaps; in leaps of about four feet, the distance of one foot from the cord is sufficient; in higher leaps, it should be from one and a half to two feet. The best plan is to have a small pit dug in front of the cord (see Plate XII. *figs.* 2 and 3), and to remove the stand from it, as the height of the leap increases; or the stand may remain at a foot and a half from the pit, and the learner be taught to make all the leaps from it. The spring is made with one foot, at the distance of two, three, four, or five feet from the plant of the pole. If the leaper keep the left hand lowest, he must spring with the left foot, and vice versa.

Four. The swing upward is effected by the force of the spring, the support of the lower, and the pull of the upper hand; but principally by the propulsion of the run, which being suddenly modified by the fixing of the pole, has its horizontal direction changed into a slanting ascent, and carries the body of the leaper over the cord. The leaper must carefully observe that the spring of the foot, and the plant of the pole, be in the direction of the preparatory run.

Five. The turning of the body during the swinging upward, is necessary. When the leaper is going to spring, he has his face turned towards the object of the leap, as in Plate XII. *fig.* 1; but as his feet swing, his body turns round the pole. When his feet have passed over the other side of the cord, the head is still considerably on this side: the leaper then appears as in *fig.* 2. Speedily, the middle of his body is on the other side of the cord, and he begins the descent, as in *fig.* 3. It would be impossible to descend in this position otherwise than with his face directed to the place where the leap was commenced.

Six. The quitting of the pole during the leap is effected by giving it a push with one hand, at the moment of greatest height, and this causes it to fall on the inner side of the cord.

Seven. The carrying of the pole over the cord is more difficult. The leaper must then raise the pole a little from the ground at the moment of beginning the descent, and instantly elevate the lower part of it with the lowest hand, and depress the upper part with the other; the consequence being, that, at the descent, the lower end of the pole will point upward, and the upper end downward. This should be practised first in low leaps.

Eight. The descent depends entirely upon the manner in which the leap is made: if the leap be perfect, the descent will be so. The usual fault in descending is, that the leaper, having passed the cord, falls to the ground almost perpendicularly instead of obliquely. In the overleaf figure, *a* is the place whence the spring is made, *c* the section of the cord, *b* the position of the leaper over it, *d* his right, and *e* his wrong descent. The latter is faulty because it throws him so much out of balance, that in order not to fall backward, he must run backward to *d*. If, on the contrary, he descends in proper balance to the ground, he moves not an inch from the spot where his feet alight; and this complete rest following the descent is the sign of a perfect leap. The descent, as already explained, must take place upon the balls of the toes, and with a sinking of the knees. The position of the body is sufficiently explained by Plate XII.

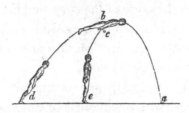

figs. 1, 2, and 3; but many learn to swing the legs so well as to raise them, during the highest part of the leap, considerably above the head. Order of exercises in the high leap, to be very gradually attempted:

1. The height of the hips.
2. That of the pit of the stomach.
3. That of the chin.
4. That of the crown of the head.
5. That of the points of the fingers – that is, as high as the latter can reach.

In performing these leaps, the pole is parted with. Many more may form a repetition of the preceding, with this difference, that the leaper carries the pole over with him. A similar number may repeat the first, except that the leaper, between the spring and descent, makes a complete turn round the pole, so as again to bring his face in the direction of the leap. This enlarged turn is rendered easier by leaping a little higher than the cord requires.

THE LONG LEAP WITH A POLE

This leap is the most useful, being applicable almost everywhere; and particularly in a country intersected with small

rivers, ditches, &c. It should be first practised over a ditch
about three feet deep, eight feet broad at one end, and
about twenty-one feet at the other, and of any convenient
length. In this exercise, the pole should be rather stronger
and longer than in the preceding one – depending, however, on the length of the leap, and the height of the bank it
is made from. The usual length is from ten to thirteen feet.

The handling of the pole is the same as in the high leap.
The preparatory run is rapid, in proportion to the length
of the leap. The spring takes place as in the preceding exercise. The swing is also the same, except that the curve of
the leap is wider. The turning of the body may likewise be
similar, but it is convenient to make only a quarter turn.
In the descent, the hand presses more upon the pole; and
the feet are stretched out to reach the opposite bank, as in
Plate XIII. *fig*. 1, in which the leaper is descending. Another
method of leaping a river, is to force the body up so high by
the pressure of the hands (of which one rests upon the end
of the pole, or very near it) as to swing over the top of the
pole, and allow it to pass between the legs when descending
(Plate XIII. *fig*. 2).

Try the following:

1. The leap of two lengths of the body.
2. That of three lengths of the body.
3. That of four lengths of the body.
4. Persons of equal strength try to outleap
   one another.

The lengths of 18, 20, 22, and 24 feet are frequently done
by practised leapers.

PLATE XIII

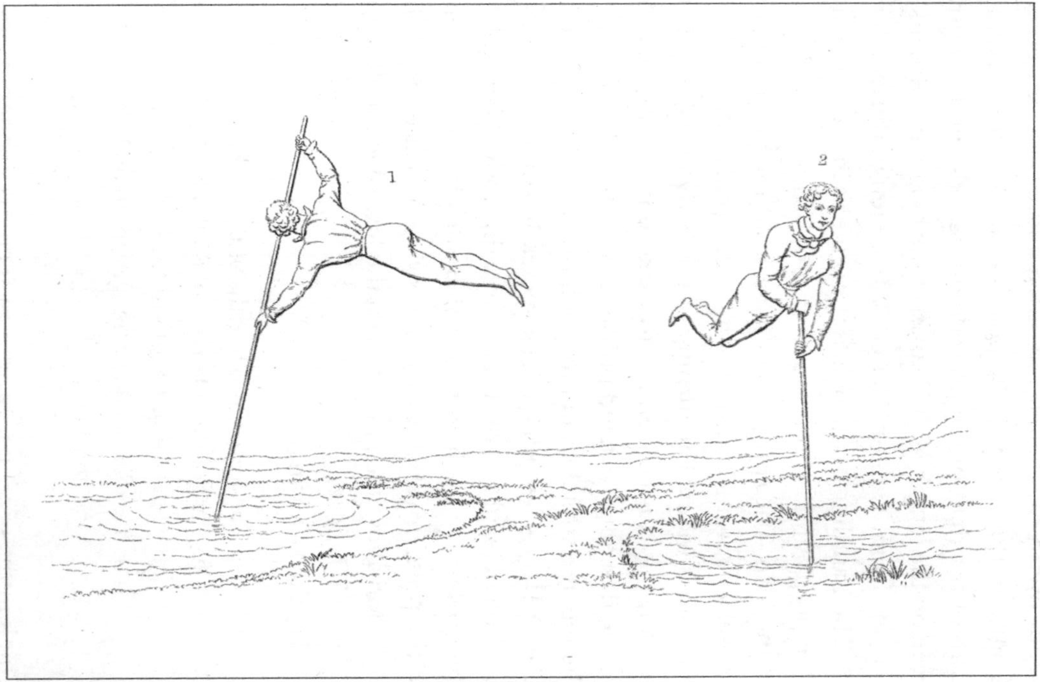

POLE LEAPING

THE DEEP LEAP WITH A POLE

Here neither the preparatory run nor the spring occur: there is nothing which requires the exertion of the lower members. The use of the hands and arms, however, is peculiarly requisite, as well as a little of the art of balancing. The leaper fixes the pole, at a convenient distance from the place where he stands, in a chasm, ditch, or river, having one bank high, and the opposite one low. Seizing it with both hands in the usual way, he slips along it lower and lower; the whole weight of his body, at last, resting upon it. Thus, if the depth is considerable, as two lengths of the body, he may slide so far down upon it, that his head appears slanting downward. In this position, he makes a slight push against the bank, or merely quits it, with his feet, which he swings by the side of the pole to the opposite bank. Here, also, the descent is performed upon the balls of the toes, with bending of the knees. The principal advantage in this leap lies in the art of supporting the body, without tottering; and for this purpose, it is absolutely necessary that the feet should be stretched out far from each other, in an angular form, otherwise the balance might be lost. The best way of practising this is by a flight of steps.

To the exercise of the abdominal members, these leaps unite a strong action of the muscles of the thorax, arms, and forearms, and even of those of the palms of the hand. The body is only half impelled by the abdominal members; but this impulse is rendered complete by considerable effort on the part of the thoracic members. The latter, in the vertical leap, being supported by the narrow and moveable base afforded by the pole, assist greatly in raising the body, and even keep it a moment suspended for the legs to pass over (if the object to be cleared is very high) before they allow the body to obey the force of gravity which carries it down.

This exercise communicates what is termed great lightness to the body, and great suppleness – that is to say, great relative strength of the abdominal members; and it also develops the superior members. It is good for lymphatic temperaments and young persons, but it should not be indulged in immediately after meals. It may occasion accidents of the brain and spinal marrow, unless all the articulations are bent on returning to the ground.

BALANCING

BALANCING is the art of preserving the stability of the body upon a narrow or a moving surface. The balancing bar consists of a round and tapering pole, supported horizontally, about three feet from the ground, by upright posts, one at its thicker extremity, and another about the middle, between the parts of which it may be raised or lowered by means of an iron peg passing through holes in their sides. The unsupported end of the bar wavers, of course, when stepped upon (Plate XIV).

The upper surface of the bar being smooth in dry weather, the soles of the shoes should be damped; the ground about the bar should consist of sand, and the exercises be cautiously performed.

PLATE XIV

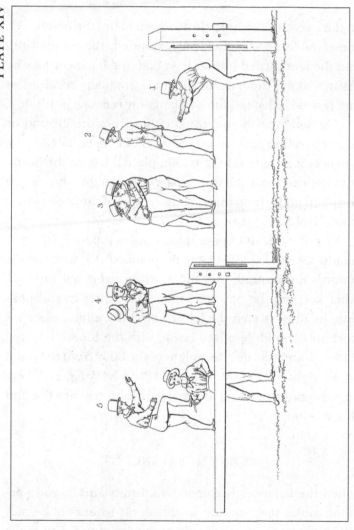

BALANCING

POSITION AND ACTION IN BALANCING

In this exercise, the head should be held up, the body erect, the shoulders back, the arms extended, the hands shut, and the feet turned outward. At first, the balancer may be assisted along the bar; but he must gradually receive less and less aid, till at last the assistant only remains by his side.

The pole may be mounted either from the ground or from the riding position on the beam. In the latter case, the balancer may raise the right foot, place it flat on the beam, with the heel near the upper part of the thigh, and rise on the point of the foot, carrying the weight of the body before him (Plate XIV. *fig.* 1).

In this case, the beam must not be touched with the hands; the left leg must hang perpendicularly, with the toe towards the ground, and the arms be stretched forward. After keeping the balance for some minutes in this position, he must stretch the left leg out before him, place his heel on the middle of the beam, with the toe well turned outward, and transfer the weight of the body from the point of the right foot to the left heel (Plate XIV. *fig.* 2). These steps he must perform alternately, till he reaches the end of the beam.

TURNS IN BALANCING

When the balancer is able to walk firmly and in good position along the bar, and to spring off whenever he may lose his balance, he may attempt to turn round, first at the broad, then at the narrow end, and to return. He may next try to go backward.

In accomplishing this, it is no longer the heel, but the tip of the toes, which receives the weight; the leg which hangs being stretched backward, with the hip, knee, and heel forming a right angle, till the toes, by a transverse motion, are so placed on the middle of the beam, that the balancer can safely transfer to them the whole weight of the body.

To acquire the art of passing an obstacle placed laterally, two balancers may pass each other thus: They must hold one another fast by the arms, advance breast to breast, place each his right foot close forward to that of his comrade, across the bar (Plate XIV. *fig.* 3), and turn completely round each other, by each stepping with his left foot round the right one of the other, as in Plate XIV. *fig.* 4.

To acquire the art of passing an obstacle placed inferiorly, a large stone may be laid upon the bar, or a stick may be held before the balancer, about the height of the knee (Plate XIV. *fig.* 5).

To pass over men placed upon a beam, the pupil or pupils who are astride in front lie down on the beam, which they grasp firmly by passing their arms round it. The pupil *a* (Plate XV. *fig.* 1), having to pass to the point on the beam marked *b*, places his hands on the waistband of his comrade *c*: he then leans upon his arms, and raises his body to pass forward over his comrade, opening his legs widely, so as not to touch him, till he places himself astride at *c*. He then extends his hands and arms for a second movement, places them at *b*, and leans the body well forward, as shown

in Plate XV. *fig.* 2. Being thus placed, he makes the last
movement, raises his body upon the arms to pass over his
comrade's head without touching it, which is the chief rule
of this exercise, and places himself astride upon the beam
at *b*, moving his hands immediately, and extending them to
rest at *d*. This movement being finished, he continues advancing astride, along the beam, over the others, if there be
any; raises himself to an upright position, and lies down in
his turn on the beam. This last attitude requires some care,
because the head must incline either to the right or left of
the beam, as shown in the plates, and the pupil must hold
tight to the beam with the arms and thighs, which requires
both skill and strength.

The pupil may also pass as shown in Plate XV. *fig.* 3.
This method is very easy for the person passing and indeed
more so than any other; but it is necessary that the pupil
who is in the position *b* should have learnt to raise himself
up on the beam, or know how to advance along it under-
neath, in a reversed position.

It is impossible for anyone who has not seen the carni-
vals of Venice, and other towns in Italy, to form an idea of
all the difficulties that have been surmounted in the art
of equilibrium. To acquire the art of carrying any body,
the balancer may at first walk along the bar with his hands
folded across his breast, instead of using them to balance
himself; and he may afterwards carry bodies of various
magnitudes.

To this notice of the rules by which the art of Balancing
may be best acquired, it will not be out of place to subjoin
a slight outline of its importance to all who desire to arrive

PLATE XV

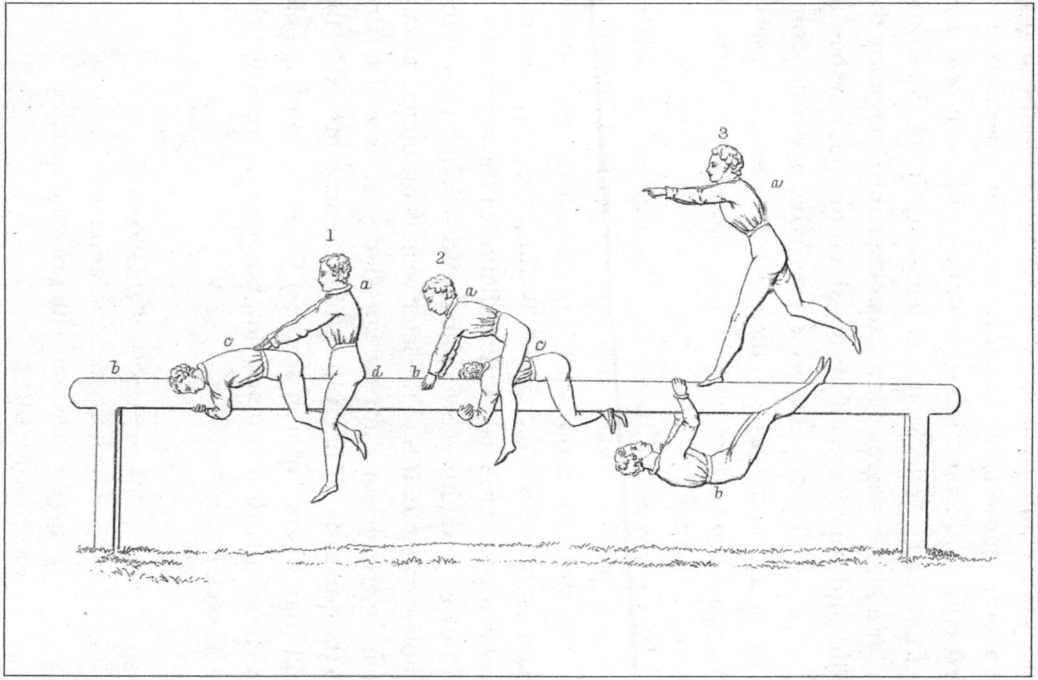

BALANCING

at excellence in any of the Manly Exercises. Motion – the source of them all – if not absolutely dependent for existence upon equilibrium, without it would be but the infancy of action – movement tottering, uncertain, powerless. The first effort of locomotion – the walk – without it possesses neither force nor decision: it is demanded in the same ratio as for a higher degree of muscular exertion, increasing the value and importance of the art which teaches how best to apply the vital energies to its service. What a wise economy is to the social, this art is to the physical system: both serve to augment our resources, by instructing us to husband them against future need.

While in every instance equilibrium adds greatly to physical power, in many it stands altogether in its stead. To the most casual observer of our usual sports, it will be manifest that this is the case in Skating; the more attentive and competent will have little difficulty in tracing its effects in Leaping, Vaulting, Swimming, and through almost the whole catalogue. It is to the later writers on horsemanship that we are indebted for the knowledge of its vital service to the equestrian. The truth of their theory is proved by the fact that, where formerly scarce a tithe of a hunting-field was found to ride to hounds, now nine-tenths are ordinarily to be seen in good places.

> ———Scouring along,
> In pleasing hurry and confusion toss'd,
> Happy the man, who with unrival'd speed
> Can pass his fellows.

CARRYING WEIGHT

THE power of raising and carrying weight is of great importance in a general view. Many advantages will be derived
from it; for besides strengthening the locomotive muscles,
upon which all our physical operations depend, it will
fortify also all the system and all the organs. All persons,
moreover, may find themselves under the necessity of rais
ing and carrying a wounded or fainting person, and may be
glad to have cultivated and acquired the power necessary to
perform such an act.

In accustoming young persons to carry burdens, they
should be taught to support what is on the back first with
one hand and then with the other; by these means the
muscles are equally exercised on each side, and acquire an
equal development. These burdens, however, must not exceed their strength; and they should be taught not to carry
on one side in preference, for fear of deforming the limbs.
There are several modes of supporting weights, and of try-
ing the amount of power possessed for this kind of exercise.

Plate XVI. *fig.* 1 represents one method. It consists
in loading the shoulders with sacks full of articles whose
weight is previously known. The position of the arms and
hands is such that the pupil can support a great weight: but
in this way he can walk but very slowly; and it is, therefore,
so far, disadvantageous.

Fig. 2, in the same plate, supports a weight by means of
a hod. This is filled with balls or stones, of which the weight
is known.

The form of the weight is of consequence. A soldier now

PLATE XVI

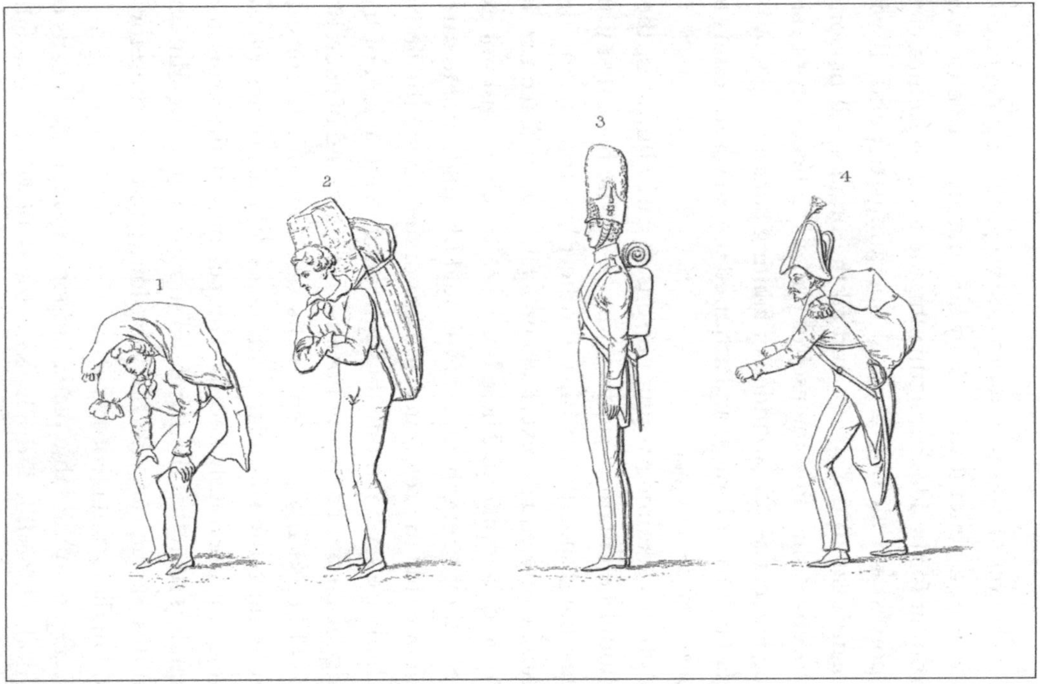

CARRYING WEIGHT

carries with ease a knapsack full of articles, and additional weight above it, because the flat shape that has been lately adopted fits the body, and lies close to the back, as in *fig.* 3, and the centre of gravity is thus very little deranged. But if the knapsack were of the old shape, very projecting and very round, as in *fig.* 4, the soldier would be forced to incline his body forward, and would not be able to carry as great a weight, nor march as long a time, in consequence of fatigue. It is for this reason, among others, desirable to extend the knowledge of the most simple rules of mechanics, because these rules are serviceable in avoiding many dangers, and diminishing the fatigue and the efforts that vacillation in the movements produces. We may make use of a hook to bear boxes or bags in addition, with the weights marked, and thus learn the carrier's strength.

Milo, says history, first carried a calf immediately after its birth, and continued to do so every day till it had reached its full size. It was said by this means that he was able to carry even the ox itself, and afterwards throw it on the ground and kill it with his fist.

Augustus the Second, King of Poland, carried a man upon his hand.

A man named Roussel, a labourer in the environs of Lisle, who on a smaller scale (being but four feet ten inches in height), was formed exactly like the Farnese Hercules, raised on his shoulders a weight of eighteen hundred pounds. He cleared a circle six feet in height with very little spring and one hundred weight in each hand. When seated on the ground, he rose up without aid, carrying two men on his arms. Equally astonishing in the strength of his loins, he took up a two hundred-weight leaning backward

over a chair. 'I have seen this remarkable man,' says Fried-
lander: 'the whole of his family are very strong: his sister
and brother are equally remarkable in this point.' It is very
striking to find in him the characteristic traits with which
antiquity depicted the ideal of bodily strength.

In the Encyclopaedia of Kruntz, vol. lxxii., we find instances of some men similar to Roussel, who lived at the
commencement of the last century. A man named Ecken-
berg raised a cannon of two thousand five hundred pounds
weight; and two strong men were unable to take from him
a stick that he held between his teeth.

In number 446 of the Bibliotheque Britannique, is to be
found a report of some trials made by a Mr Shulze, in his
manufactory, of the strength of men of different heights.
These trials show what influence an elevated stature has
upon the vertical height to which a man can raise any
weight. A short man is, in his turn, capable of employing
more force in another direction.

————————

THROWING THE DISCUS

AMONG the Greeks, throwing the discus did not form part
of the games till the eighteenth Olympiad. This exercise
consisted in throwing, as far as possible, a mass of wood or
stone, but more commonly of iron or copper, of a lenticular
form. From the testimony of ancient authors, there was no
fixed mark or butt, except the spot where the discus thrown
by the strongest of the discoboli alighted. Mercuriali has
handed down to us three engravings, in which the discus is

PLATE XVII

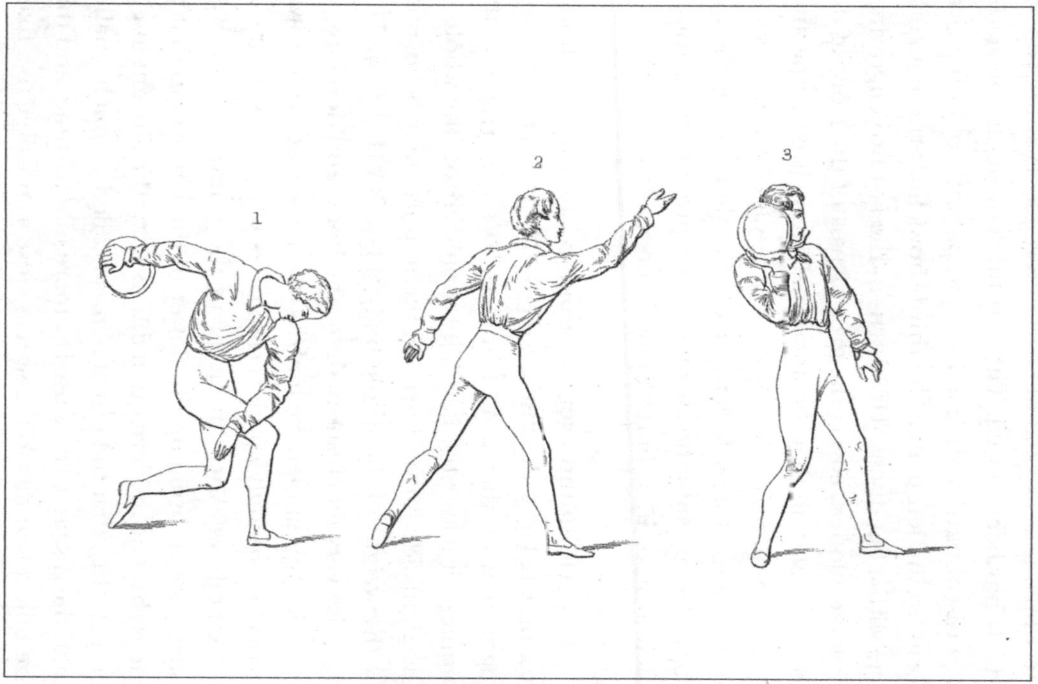

1   2   3

THROWING THE DISCUS

not of the same shape. The first engraving represents four discoboli in the act of throwing with the right hand a discus which is as thick at the circumference as at the centre, which has been bored. The second represents the statue of a discobulus holding a discus, apparently of a spherical form, in the left hand. The third shows the arm of an athlete with a flat discus. The discus in the last two engravings now mentioned, covers the greater part of the front of the forearm; and all that the ancients have written respecting this instrument, tends to show that it was of enormous size and weight. Homer tells us that the athletes threw the discus either up into the air merely as a prelude to accustom their arms to it, or horizontally when they were striving for the prize.

To perform this exercise properly, the thrower should not only balance the discus well on the right arm (supposing it to be on that arm, as in Plate XVII. *fig.* 1); but at the moment it leaves the hand, he should throw the whole of the right side forward, so that the impulse may be assisted by the weight of the whole body (Plate XVII. *fig.* 2). This exercise very much strengthens the body, and develops, in a particular manner, the limb by which the discus is thrown. It may be usefully employed in cases where it is desirable to remedy weakness in either of the arms; and it is well calculated to bring up the power of the left arm to that of the right. The modern quoit differs from the ancient discus only in this, that the instrument so called is much smaller than the discus, that its use is a mere idle pastime, and that the object is always to throw it as close as possible to a fixed mark, requiring more skill than strength.

It is evident that the discus may be heaved from above

the shoulder as well as flung from below (see Plate XVII. *fig.* 3). No exercises can excel these for the acquirement of power. They ought to be much practised with both hands. A man of moderate strength will throw a pound weight of lead a distance of 140 feet, or thereabouts.

Silex $1\frac{1}{2}$	·	·	·	126 feet
Ditto $\frac{1}{4}$	·	·	·	145 "
Brick $\frac{1}{2}$	·	·	·	160 "

CLIMBING

CLIMBING is the art of transporting the body in any direction, by the aid, in general, both of the hands and feet. The climbing-stand consists of two strong poles, about fifteen feet high, and from fifteen to twenty-five feet distant, which are firmly fixed on the ground, and support a beam strongly fastened to them. One pole is two inches and a half in diameter; the other, which serves as a mast, should be considerably thicker; and both serve the purpose of climbing. To the beam are attached other implements of climbing: viz. a ladder, an inclined board, an upright pole, a mast, an inclined pole, a horizontal bar, a rope ladder, an upright, an inclined, and a level rope (Plate XVIII).

KINDS OF CLIMBING

Climbing on fixed bodies should first be practised.

The Ladder

Exercises on the ladder may be practised in the following ways:

    1. By ascending and descending as usual.
    2. With one hand, carrying something in the other.
    3. Without using the hands.
    4. Passing another on the front of the ladder, or
       swinging to the back, to let another pass.

The Inclined Board

This should be rather rough, about two feet broad, and two inches thick. To climb it, it is necessary to seize both sides with the hands, and to place the feet flat in the middle, the inclination of the board being diminished with the progress of the pupil.

At first, it may form with the ground an angle of about thirty degrees; and the climber should not go more than half-way up. This angle may gradually be augmented to a right angle, or the direction of the board may be made perpendicular. When the board is thus little or not at all inclined, the body must be much curved inward, and the legs thrust up, so that the higher one is nearly even with the hand. In descending, small and quick steps are necessary.

The Upright Pole

The upright pole should be about two inches and a half in diameter, perfectly smooth and free from splinters.

The position of the climber is shown in Plate XVIII. *fig.* 1, where nothing touches the pole except the feet, legs, knees, and hands. He grasps as high as possible with both hands, raises himself by bending the body and drawing his legs up the pole, holds fast by them, extends the body, again grasps higher up with his hands, and continues the same use of the legs and arms. The descent is performed by sliding down with the legs, and scarcely touching with the hands, as in Plate XVIII. *fig.* 2.

The Mast

This is more difficult, as it cannot be grasped with the hands; and it consequently should not be practised until the climber is expert in the previous exercises. The position of the legs is the same as for the pole; but, instead of grasping the mast, the climber lays hold of his left arm with his right hand, or the reverse, and clings to the mast with the whole body, as in Plate XVIII. *fig.* 3.

The Slant Pole

This must be at least three inches thick; and as, in this exercise, the hands bear more of the weight than in climbing the upright pole, it should not be attempted until expertness in the other is acquired.

The Horizontal, or Slightly Inclined Bar

This may be about two inches wide at top, from ten to fifteen feet long, and supported by two posts, respectively six and seven feet high. The climber must grasp with both hands as high a part of the bar as he can reach, and, with arms extended, support his own weight as long as possible. He must next endeavour to bend the elbows so much, that one shoulder remains close under the bar, as seen in

Plate XVIII. *fig.* 4. Or he may place both hands on the same side, and draw himself up so far as to see over it, keeping the legs and feet close and extended.

He may then hang with his hands fixed on both sides, near to each other, having the elbows much bent, the upper parts of the arms close to the body, and one shoulder close under the bar; he may lower the head backward, and may, at the same time, raise the feet to touch each other over the bar (Plate XVIII. *fig.* 5). In the last position, he may move the hands one before the other, forward or backward, and may either slide the feet along the bar, or alternately change them like the hands, and retain a similar hold.

Hanging also by the hands alone, as in Plate XVIII. *fig.* 6, he moves them either forward or backward, keeping the arms firm, and the feet close and extended. Or he may place himself in front of the bar, hanging by both hands, and move laterally. Being likewise in front of the bar, with his hands resting upon it, as in Plate XVIII. *fig.* 7, he may move along the bar either to the right or left. In the position of Plate XVIII. *fig.* 5, the climber may endeavour to sit upon the bar, for instance, on the right side, by taking hold with the right knee-joint, grasping firmly with the right hand, and bringing the left armpit over the bar. The riding position is thus easily obtained. From the riding position, he may, by supporting himself with one thigh, turn towards the front of the bar, allowing the leg of the other side to hang down; and he may then very easily move along the bar sideways, by raising his body with his hands placed laterally on the bar.

The Rope Ladder

This should have several rundles to spread it out, and

ought, in all respects, to be so constructed, as not to twist and entangle. The only difficulty here is that, as it hangs perpendicularly, and is flexible, its steps are liable to be pushed forward, and in that case, the body is thrown into an oblique position, and the whole weight falls on the hands. To prevent this, the climber must keep the body stretched out and upright (Plate XVIII. *fig.* 8).

The Upright Rope

In this exercise, the securing of the rope may be effected in various ways. In the first method, shown in Plate XVIII. *fig.* 9, the hands and feet alone are employed. The feet are crossed; the rope passes between them, and is held fast by their pressure; the hands then grasp higher; the feet are drawn up; they are again applied to the rope; and the same process is repeated. In the second, which is the sailor's method, shown at Plate XVIII. *fig.* 10, the rope passes from the hands, generally along the right thigh, just above the knee; winds round the inside of the thigh, under the knee-joint, over the outside of the leg, and across the instep, whence it hangs loose; and the climber, by treading with the left foot upon that part of the rope where it crosses the right one, is firmly supported. This mode of climbing requires the right leg and foot to be so managed that the rope keeps its proper winding whenever it is quitted by the left foot. In descending, to prevent injury, the hands must be lowered alternately.

To rest upon the upright rope, the climber must swing the right foot around the rope, so as to wind it three or four times round the leg; must turn it, by means of the left foot, once or twice round the right one, of which the toes

PLATE XVIII

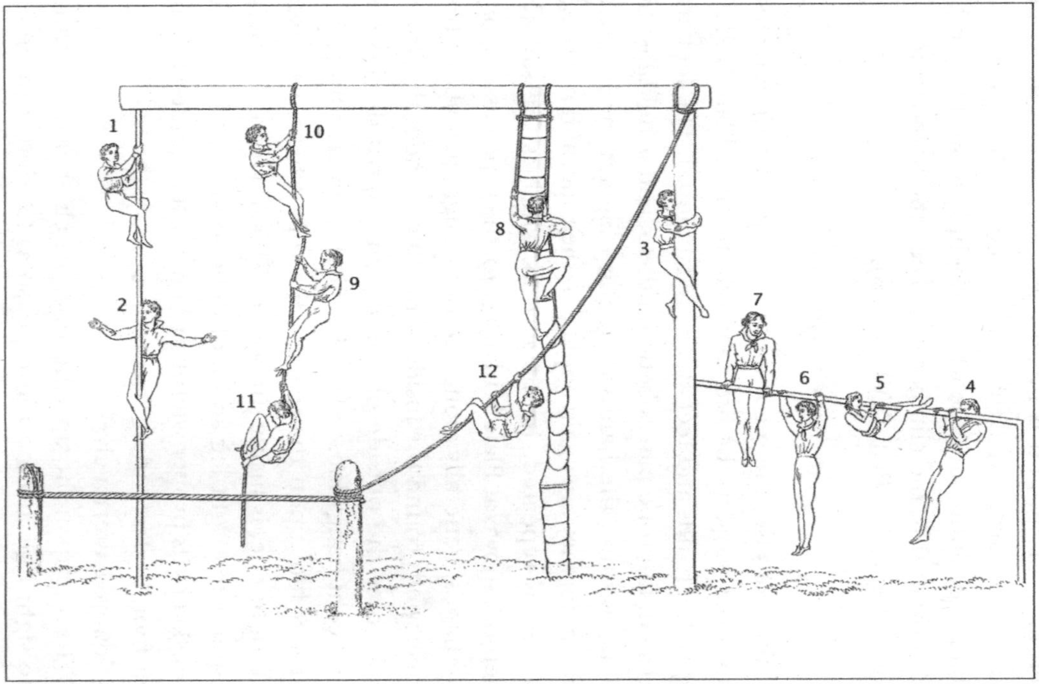

CLIMBING

are to be bent upward; and must tread firmly with the left foot upon the last winding. Or, to obtain a more perfect rest, he may lower his hands along the rope, as in Plate XVIII. *fig.* 11, hold with the right hand, stoop, grasp with the left the part of the rope below the feet, raise it and himself again, and wind it round his shoulders, &c., until he is firmly supported.

The Oblique Rope

The climber must fix himself to the rope, as in Plate XVIII. *fig.* 12, and advance the hands along it, as already directed. The feet may move along the rope alternately; or one leg, hanging over the rope, may slide along it; or, which is best, the sole of one foot may be laid upon the rope, and the other leg across its instep, so that the friction is not felt.

The Level Rope

This may have its ends fastened to posts of equal heights; and the same exercises may be performed upon it.

Climbing Trees

In attempting this exercise, the type of wood and strength of the branches must be considered. Summer is the best time for practising it, as withered branches are then most easily discerned; and even then it is best to climb low trees, until some experience is acquired. As the surface of branches is smooth, or moist and slippery, the hands must never for a moment be relaxed.

SKATING

Skating is the art of balancing the body, while, by the impulse of each foot alternately, it moves rapidly upon the ice.

CONSTRUCTION OF THE SKATE

The wood of the skate should be slightly hollowed, so as to adapt it to the ball of the foot; and, as the heel of the boot must be thick enough to admit the peg, it may be well to lower the wood of the skate corresponding to the heel, so as to permit the foot to regain that degree of horizontal position which it would otherwise lose by the height of the heel; for the more of the foot that is in contact with the skate, the more firmly will these be attached. As the tread of the skate should correspond, as nearly as possible, with that of the foot, the wood should be of the same length as the boot or shoe; the irons of good steel, and well secured in the wood.

These should pass beyond the screw at the heel, nearly as far as the wood itself; but the bow of the iron should not project much beyond the tread.

If the skate project much beyond the wood, the whole foot, and more especially its hind part, must be raised considerably from the ice when the front or bow of the skate is brought to bear upon it; and, as the skater depends upon this part for the power of his stroke, it is evident that that must be greatly diminished by the general distance of the foot from the ice. In short, if the skate be too long, the stroke will be feeble, and the back of the leg painfully cramped: if it be too short, the footing will be proportionally unsteady and tottering.

As the position of the person in the act of skating is never vertical, and is sometimes very much inclined, and as considerable exertion of the muscles of the leg is requisite to keep the ankle stiff, this ought to be relieved by the lowness of the skates. Seeing, then, that the closer the foot is to the ice, the less is the strain on the ankle, it is clear that the foot ought to be brought as near to the ice as possible, without danger of bringing the sole of the shoe in contact with it, while traversing on the edge of the skate. The best height is about three-quarters of an inch, and the iron about a quarter of an inch thick.

The grooved or fluted skate, if ever useful, is of service only to boys, or very light persons, whose weight is not sufficient to catch the ice in a hard frost. It certainly should never be used by a person who is heavier than a boy of thirteen or fourteen years of age usually is, because the sharp edge too easily cuts into the ice, and prevents figuring. Fluted skates, indeed, are even dangerous: for the snow or ice cuttings are apt to collect and consolidate in the grooves, till the skater is raised from the edge of his skate, and thrown.

In the general inclination of the foot in skating, no edge can have greater power than that of rectangular shape: the tendency of its action is downward, cutting through rather than sliding on the surface; and greater hold than this is unnecessary. The irons of skates should be kept well and sharply ground. This ought to be done across the stone, so as to give the bottom of the skate so slight a concavity as to be imperceptible, which ensures an edge whose angle is not greater than right. Care must be taken that one edge is not higher than the other; so that when the skate is placed upon an even surface, it may stand quite perpendicularly. The wear of the iron not being great with a beginner, one grinding will generally last him through an ordinary winter's skating on clean ice.

The bottom of the iron should be a little curved; for, if perfectly straight, it would be capable of describing only a straight line, whereas the skater's progress must be circular, because, in order to bring the edge to bear, the body must be inclined, and inclination can be preserved only in circular motion. This curve of the iron should be part of a circle, whose radius is about two feet. That shape enables the skater to turn his toe or heel outward or inward with facility.

A screw would have a firmer hold than a mere peg in the hole of the boot; but, as it is less easily removed, skaters generally prefer the peg. The skater should be careful not to bore a larger hole in the heel than is sufficient to admit the peg. The more simple the fastenings of the skate the better. The two straps – namely, the cross strap over the toe, and the heel strap – cannot be improved, unless perhaps by passing one strap through the three bores, and so making it serve for both.

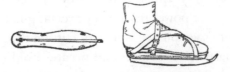

Before going on the ice, the young skater must learn to tie on the skates, and may also learn to walk with them easily in a room, balancing alternately on each foot.

DRESS OF THE SKATER

A skater's dress should be as close and unencumbered as possible. Large skirts get entangled with his own limbs, or those of the persons who pass near him; and all fullness of dress is exposed to the wind. Loose trousers, frocks, and more especially great-coats, must be avoided; and indeed, by wearing additional under-clothing, they can always be dispensed with.

As the exercise of skating produces perspiration, flannel next to the chest, shoulders, and loins is necessary to avoid the evils produced by sudden chills in cold weather. The best dress is what is called a dress-coat, buttoned, tight pantaloons, and laced boots (having the heel no higher than is necessary for the peg), which hold the foot tightly and steadily in its place, as well as give the best support to the ankle; for it is of no use to draw the straps of the skate hard, if the boot or the shoe be loose.

PRELIMINARY AND GENERAL DIRECTIONS

Either very rough or very smooth ice should be avoided. The person who for the first time attempts to skate, must not trust to a stick. He may make a friend's hand his support, if he require one; but that should be soon relinquished, in order to balance himself. He will probably scramble about for half an hour or so, till he begins to find out where the edge of his skate is.

The beginner must be fearless, but not violent; nor even in a hurry. He should not let his feet get far apart, and keep his heels still nearer together. He must keep the ankle of the foot on the ice quite firm; not attempting to gain the edge of the skate by bending it, because the right mode of getting to either edge is by the inclination of the whole body in the direction required; and this inclination should be made fearlessly and decisively.

The leg which is on the ice should be kept perfectly straight; for, though the knee must be somewhat bent at the time of striking, it must be straightened as quickly as possible without any jerk. The leg which is off the ice should also be kept straight, though not stiff, having an easy but slight play, the toe pointing downward, and the heel within from six to twelve inches of the other.

The learner must not look down at the ice, nor at his feet, to see how they perform. He may at first incline his body a little forward, for safety, but hold his head up, and see where he goes, his person erect, and his face rather elevated than otherwise.

When once off, he must bring both feet up together, and strike again, as soon as he finds himself steady enough, rarely allowing both feet to be on the ice together. The position of the arms should be easy and varied; one being always more raised than the other, this elevation being alternate, and the change corresponding with that of the legs; that is, the right arm being raised as the right leg is put down, and vice versa, so that the arm and leg of the same side may not be raised together.

The face must be always turned in the direction of the line intended to be described. Hence, in backward skating, the head will be inclined much over the shoulder; in forward skating, but slightly. All sudden and violent action

must be avoided. Stopping may be caused by slightly bending the knees, drawing the feet together, inclining the body
forward, and pressing on the heels. It may also be caused
by turning short to the right or left, the foot on the side to
which we turn being rather more advanced, and supporting part of the weight.

THE ORDINARY RUN, OR INSIDE EDGE FORWARD

The first attempt of the beginner is to walk, and this walk
shortly becomes a sliding gait, done entirely on the inside
edge of the skate.

The first impulse is to be gained by pressing the inside
edge of one skate against the ice, and advancing with the
opposite foot. To effect this, the beginner must bring the
feet nearly together, turn the left somewhat out, place the
right a little in advance and at right angles with it, lean
forward with the right shoulder, and at the same time move
the right foot onwards, and press sharply, or strike the ice
with the inside edge of the left skate, care being taken instantly to throw the weight on the right foot (Plate XIX.
fig. 1). While thus in motion, the skater must bring up the
left foot nearly to a level with the other, and may for the
present proceed a short way on both feet.

He must next place the left foot in advance in its turn,
bring the left shoulder forward, inclining to that side, strike
from the inside edge of the right skate, and proceed as
before.

Finally, this motion has only to be repeated on each
foot alternately, gradually keeping the foot from which
he struck longer off the ice, till he has gained sufficient

PLATE XIX

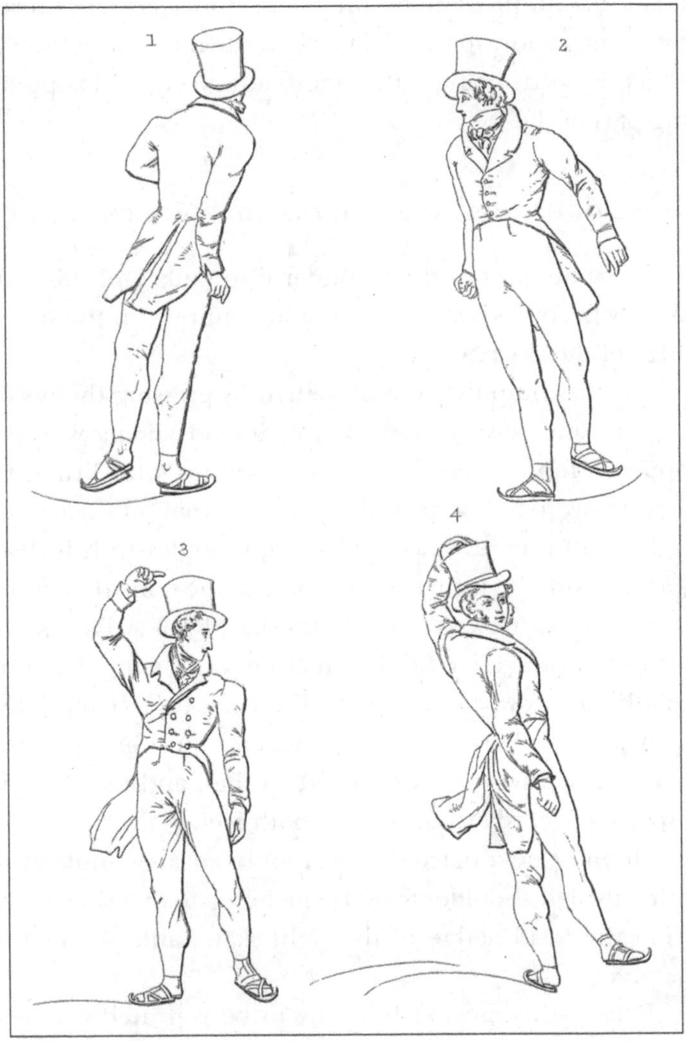

command of himself to keep it off altogether, and is able to strike directly from one to the other, without at any time having them both on the ice together. Having practised this till he has gained some degree of firmness and power, and a command of his balance, he may proceed to:

THE FORWARD ROLL, OR OUTSIDE EDGE

This is commonly reckoned the first step to figure skating, as, when it is once effected, the rest follows with ease. The impulse is gained in the same manner as for the ordinary run; but, to get on the outside edge of the right foot, the moment that foot is in motion, the skater must advance the left shoulder, throw the right arm back, look over the right shoulder, and incline the whole person boldly and decisively on that side, keeping the left foot suspended behind (Plate XIX. *fig.* 2).

As he proceeds, he must bring the left foot past the inside of the right, with a slight jerk, which produces an opposing balance of the body; the right foot must quickly press, first on the outside of the heel, then on the inside, or its toe; the left foot must be placed down in front, before it is removed more than about eight or ten inches from the other foot; and, by striking outside to the left, giving at the same moment a strong push with the inside of the right toe, the skater passes from right to left, inclining to the left side, in the same manner as he did to the right. He then continues to change from left to right, and from right to left, in the same manner. At first he should not remain long upon one leg, nor scruple occasionally to put the other down to assist; and throughout he must keep himself erect, leaning most on the heel.

The Dutch travelling roll is done on the outside edge forward, in a manner just represented, except that there is described a small segment of a very large circle, thus:

diverging from the straight line no more than is requisite to keep the skate on its edge.

The cross roll on figure 8 is also done on the outside edge forward. This is only the completion of the circle on the outside edge; and it is performed by crossing the legs, and striking from the outside instead of the inside edge. In order to do this, as the skater draws to the close of the stroke on his right leg, he must throw the left quite across it, which will cause him to press hard on the outside of the right skate, from which he must immediately strike, at the same time throwing back the left arm, and looking over the left shoulder, to bring him well upon the outside of that skate. By completing the circle in this manner on each leg, the 8 is formed:

each circle being small, complete, and well-formed, before the foot is changed.

The Mercury figure is merely the outside and inside forward succeeding each other on the same leg alternately, by which a serpentine line is described, thus:

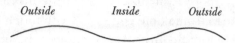

Outside   *Inside*   *Outside*

This is skated with the force and rapidity gained by a run. When the run is complete, and the skater on the outside edge, his person becomes quiescent, in the attitude of Mercury, having the right arm advanced and much raised, the face turned over the right shoulder, and the left foot off the ice, a short distance behind the other, turned out and pointed.

FIGURE OF THREE,
OR INSIDE EDGE BACKWARD

This figure is formed by turning from the outside edge forward to the inside edge backward on the same foot. The head of the 3 is formed like the half circle, on the heel of the outside edge; but when the half circle is complete, the skater leans suddenly forward, and rests on the same toe inside, and a backward motion, making the tail of the 3, is the consequence. The figure described by the right leg should be nearly in the form of No. 1; and on the left leg should be reversed, and resemble No. 2.

1   2

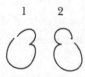

At first, the skater should not throw himself quite so hard as hitherto on the outside forward, in order that he may be able the more easily to change to the inside back. He may also be for some time contented with much less than a semicircle before he turns. Having done this, and brought the left leg nearly up to the other, he must not pass it on in advance, as he would to complete a circle, but throw it gently off sidewise, at the same moment turning the face from the right to the left shoulder, and giving the whole person a slight inclination to the left side. These motions throw the skater upon the inside of his skate; but as the first impulse should still retain most of its force, he continues to move on the inside back, in a direction so little different, that his first impulse loses little by the change (Plate XIX. fig. 3).

If unable to change the edge by this method, the skater may assist himself by slightly and gently swinging the arm and leg outward, so as to incline the person to a rotary motion. This swing, however, must be corrected as soon as the object is attained; and it must generally be observed that the change from edge to edge is to be effected merely by the inclination of the body, not by swinging.

When the skater is able to join the ends of the 3, so as to form one side of a circle, then, by striking off in the same manner, and completing another 3, with the left leg, the combination of the two 3's will form an 8. In the first attempts, the 3 should not be made above two feet long, which he will acquire the power of doing almost imperceptibly. He may then gradually extend the size as he advances in the art.

Though, in this section, backward skating is spoken of, the term refers to the skate only, which in such case moves heel foremost, but the person of the skater moves sidewise,

the face being always turned in the direction in which he
is proceeding.

OUTSIDE EDGE BACKWARD

Here the skater, having completed the 3, and being carried
on by the first impulse, still continues his progress in the
same direction, but on the other foot, putting it down on its
outside edge, and continuing to go backward slowly.

To accomplish this, the skater, after making the 3, and
placing the outside edge of his left foot on the ice, should
at once turn his face over the right shoulder, raise his right
foot from the ice, and throw back his right arm and shoulder (Plate XIX. *fig.* 4). If, for awhile, he is unable readily to
raise that foot which has made the 3, and leave himself on
the outside of the other skate, he may keep both down for
some distance, putting himself, however, in the attitude of
being on the outside only of one skate, and gradually lifting
the other off the ice as he acquires ability.

When finishing any figure, this use of both feet backward has great convenience and beauty.

Before venturing on the outside backward, the skater
ought to take care that the ice is clear of stones, reeds, &c.
and also be certain of the good quality of his irons. When
going with great force backward, the course may be deflect-
ed, so as to stop by degrees; and, whenv moving slowly, the
suspended foot may be put down in a cross direction to the
path.

Such are the four movements of which alone the skate
is capable: namely, the inside edge forward; the outside forward; the inside back; and the outside back; in which has

been seen how the impulse for the first two is gained, and how the third flows from the second, and the fourth from the third. By the combination of these elements of skating, and the variations with which they succeed each other, are formed all the evolutions in this art.

The Double Three is that combination in which the skates are brought from the inside back of the first 3, to the outside forward of the second. Here the skater, after having completed one 3, and being on the inside back, must bring the whole of the left side forward, particularly the leg, till it is thrown almost across the right, on which he is skating. This action brings him once more to the outside forward, from which he again turns to the inside back. While he is still in motion on the second inside back of the right leg, he must strike on the left, and repeat the same on that.

It is at first enough to do two 3's perfectly and smoothly. Their number from one impulse may be increased as the skater gains steadiness and skill; the art of accomplishing this being to touch as lightly as possible on each side of the skate successively, so that the first impulse may be preserved and made the most of.

The Back Roll is a means of moving from one foot to another.

Suppose the skater to have put himself on the outside back edge of the left leg, with considerable impulse, by means of the 3 performed on the right. He must not bear hard on the edge, for the object is to change it, and take up the motion on the right foot; this is effected by throwing the left arm and shoulder back, and turning the face to look over them. Having brought the inside of his left skate to bear on the ice, he must immediately strike from it to the outside back of the other, by pressing it into the ice as forcibly as he can at the toe. Having thus been brought to the backward roll on the right foot, he repeats the same with it.

The Back Cross Roll is done by changing the balance of the body, to move from one foot to the other, in the same manner as for the back roll. The stroke is from the outside instead of the inside edge of the skate; the edge on which he is skating not being changed, but the right foot, which is off the ice, being crossed at the back of the left, and put down, and the stroke taken at the same moment, from the outside edge of the left skate, at the toe. As in the back roll of both forms, the strokes are but feeble; the skater may, from time to time, renew his impulse as he finds occasion, by commencing anew with the 3.

The Large Outside Backward Roll is attained by a run, when the skater, having gained all the impulse he can, strikes on the outside forward of the right leg, turns the 3, and immediately puts down the left on the outside back. He then, without further effort, flies rapidly over the ice; the left arm being raised, the head turned over the right shoulder, and the right foot turned out and pointed.

It must be evident that the elements described may be combined and varied infinitely. Hence waltz and quadrille skating &c., which may be described as combinations of 3's, outside backward &c. These are left to the judgment of the skater, and his skill in the art.

In the North it is common to travel in skates on the gulfs and rivers; and, with a favourable wind, they go faster than vessels. It is a kind of flight, for they only touch the ground in a very slight thin line. As to feats in skating, we are told that the Frieslander, who is generally a skilful skater, often goes for a long time at the rate of fifteen miles an hour. In 1801, two young women, going thirty miles in two hours, won the prize in a skating race at Groningen. In 1821, a Lincolnshire man, for a wager of 100 guineas, skated one mile within two seconds of three minutes.

DANGERS IN SKATING

If the chest be irritable, it is neither salutary nor easy to skate against the wind. In countries where these exercises are general, inflammations of the chest are very common in winter. Skating sometimes exposes a person to much danger. If the skater finds that he cannot get away from rotten ice, he must crawl over it on his hands and knees, in order to reduce his weight on the supporting points. If he fall on it at length, he must roll away from it towards ice more firm. If he fall into a hole, he must extend his arms horizontally over the edges of the unbroken ice, and only tread water till a ladder or a plank is pushed towards him, or a rope is thrown for his hold.

TREATMENT RECOMMENDED IN THE CASE OF DROWNED PERSONS

CAUTIONS – 1. Lose no time. 2. Avoid all rough usage. 3. Never hold the body up by the feet. 4. Never roll the body on casks. 5. Nor rub the body with salt or spirits. 6. Nor inject tobacco-smoke or infusion of tobacco.

RESTORATIVE MEANS IF APPARENTLY DROWNED – Send quickly for medical assistance; but do not delay the following means.

I. Convey the body carefully, with the head and shoulders supported in a raised position, to the nearest house.

II. Strip the body, and rub it dry; then wrap it in hot blankets and place it in a warm bed in a warm chamber.

III. Wipe and cleanse the mouth and nostrils.

IV. In order to restore the natural warmth of the body:

1. Move a heated covered warming-pan over the back and spine.

2. Put bladders or bottles of hot water, or heated bricks, to the pit of the stomach, the arm-pits, between the thighs, and to the soles of the feet.

3. Foment the body with hot flannels; but, if possible,

4. Immerse the body in a warm bath, as hot as the hand can bear without pain, as this is preferable to the other means for restoring warmth.

5. Rub the body briskly with the hand; do not, however, suspend the use of the other means at the same time.

V. In order to restore breathing, introduce the pipe of a common bellows (where the apparatus of the Society is not at hand) into one nostril, carefully closing the other and the mouth: at the same time, draw downward and push gently backward the upper part of the windpipe, to allow a more free admission of air: blow the bellows gently in order to inflate the lungs, till the breast be a little raised: the mouth and nostrils should then be set free, and a moderate pressure should be made with the hand upon the chest. Repeat this process till life appears.

VI. Electricity should be employed early by a medical assistant.

VII. Inject into the stomach, by means of an elastic tube and syringe, half a pint of warm brandy and water, or wine and water.

VIII. Apply sal-volatile or hartshorn to the nostrils.

IF APPARENTLY DEAD FROM INTENSE COLD – Rub the body with snow, ice, or cold water. Restore warmth by slow degrees; and after some time, if necessary, employ the means recommended for the drowned. In these accidents, it is highly dangerous to apply heat too early.

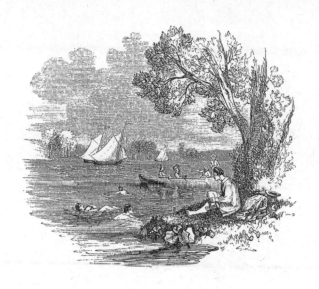

AQUATIC EXERCISES

SWIMMING

SWIMMING, considered with regard to the movements that it requires, is useful in promoting great muscular strength; but the good effects are not solely the result of the exercise that the muscles receive, but partly of the medium in which the body is moved. But the considerable increase of general force, and the tranquillizing of the nervous system produced by swimming, arise chiefly from this, that the

PLATE XX

SWIMMING – ATTITUDE

movements, in consequence of the cold and dense medium in which they take place, occasion no loss.[1]

It is easy to conceive of what utility swimming must be, where the very high state of the atmospheric temperature requires inactivity in consequence of the excessive loss caused by the slightest movement. It then becomes an exceedingly valuable resource, the only one, indeed, by which muscular weakness can be remedied, and the energy of the vital functions maintained. We must therefore regard swimming as one of the most beneficial exercises that can be taken in summer.

The ancients, particularly the Athenians, regarded swimming as indispensable; and when they wished to designate a man who was fit for nothing, they used to say, 'he cannot even swim', or 'he can neither read nor swim'. At many seaports, the art of swimming is almost indispensable; and the sailors' children are as familiar with the water as with the air. Copenhagen is perhaps the only place where sailors are trained by rules of art; and there, this exercise is more general and in greater perfection than elsewhere. It may here be observed, that it is not fear alone that prevents a man swimming. Swimming is an art that must be learnt; and fear is only an obstacle to the learning.

PREPARATORY INSTRUCTIONS AS TO ATTITUDE AND ACTION IN SWIMMING

As it is on the movements of the limbs, and a certain attitude of the body, that the power of swimming depends, its first principles may evidently be acquired out of the water.

---

1. The expression 'loss' here, is used as the result produced by increased evaporation from the pores, consequent upon violent bodily exertion.

Attitude

The head must be drawn back, and the chin elevated, the breast projected, and the back hollowed and kept steady (Plate XX. *figs*. 1 and 2). The head can scarcely be thrown too much back, or the back too much hollowed. Those who do otherwise, swim with their feet near the surface of the water, instead of having them two or three feet deep.

Action of the Hands

In the proper position of the hands, the fingers must be kept close, with the thumbs by the edge of the fore-fingers; and the hands made concave on the inside, though not so much as to diminish their size and power in swimming. The hands, thus formed, should be placed just before the breast, the wrist touching it, and the fingers pointing forward (Plate XXI. *fig*. 1).

The first elevation is formed by raising the ends of the fingers three or four inches higher than the rest of the hands. The second, by raising the outer edge of the hand two or three inches higher than the inner edge.

The formation of the hands, their first position, and their two modes of elevation, being clearly understood, the forward stroke is next made, by projecting them in that direction to their utmost extent, employing therein their first elevation, in order to produce buoyancy, but taking care the fingers do not break the surface of the water (Plate XXI. *fig*. 2). In the outward stroke of the hands, the second elevation must be employed; and, in it, they must sweep downward and outward as low as – but at a distance

PLATE XXI

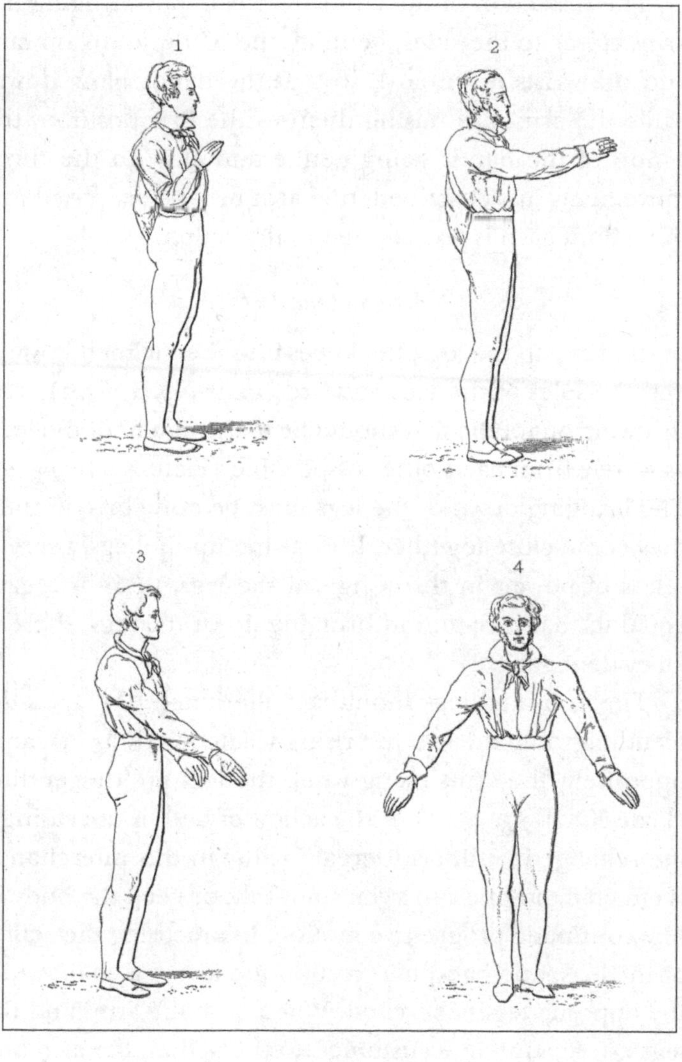

from – the hips, both laterally and anteriorly (Plate XXI. *figs*. 3 and 4).

The retraction of the hands is effected by bringing the arms closer to the sides, bending the elbow joints upward and the wrists downward, so that the hands hang down, while the arms are raising them to the first position, the action of the hands being gentle and easy. In the three movements just described, one arm may be exercised at a time, until each is accustomed to the action.

Action of the Feet

In drawing up the legs, the knees must be inclined inward, and the soles of the feet outward (Plate XXII. *fig*. 1). The throwing out of the feet should be to the extent of the legs, as widely from each other as possible (Plate XXII. *fig*. 2). The bringing down of the legs must be done briskly, until they come close together. In drawing up the legs, there is a loss of power; in throwing out the legs, there is a gain equal to that loss; and in bringing down the legs, there is an evident gain.

The arms and legs should act alternately; the arms descending while the legs are rising (Plate XXII. *fig*. 3); and, oppositely, the arms rising while the legs are descending (Plate XXII. *fig*. 4). Thus the action of both is unceasingly interchanged; and, until great facility in this interchange is effected, no one can swim smoothly, or keep the body in one continued progressive motion. In practising the action of the legs, one hand may rest on the top of a chair, while the opposite leg is exercised. When both the arms and the legs are separately accustomed to the action, the arm and leg of the same side may be exercised together.

PLATE XXII

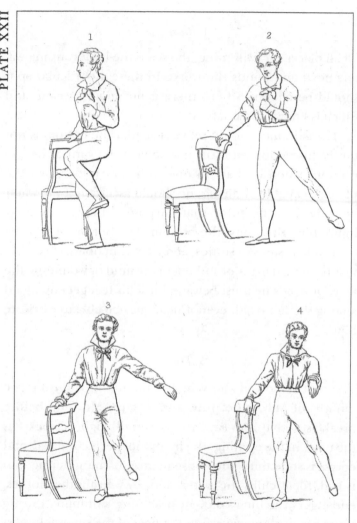

PLACE AND TIME FOR SWIMMING

Place

Of all places for swimming, the sea is the best; running waters next; and ponds the worst. In these a particular spot should be chosen, where there is not much stream, and which is known to be safe.

The swimmer should make sure that the bottom is not out of his depth; and, on this subject, he cannot be too cautious when he has no one with him who knows the place. If capable of diving, he should ascertain if the water be sufficiently deep for that purpose, otherwise, he may injure himself against the bottom. The bottom should be of gravel, or smooth stones, and free from holes, so that he may be in no danger of sinking in the mud or wounding the feet. Of weeds he must beware; for if his feet get entangled among them, no aid, even if near, may be able to extricate him.

Time

The best season of the year for swimming is during the months of May, June, July, and August. Morning before breakfast – that is to say, from seven till eight o'clock – is the time. In the evening, the hair is not perfectly dried, and coryza is sometimes the consequence. Bathing during rain is bad, for it chills the water, and, by wetting the clothes, endangers catching cold. In practising swimming during those hours of the day when the heat of the sun is felt most sensibly, if the hair be thick, it should be kept constantly wet; if the head be bald, it must be covered with a handker-chief, and frequently wetted.

It is advisable not to enter the water before digestion is finished. The danger in this case arises less from the violent movements which generally disorder digestion, than from the impression produced by the medium in which these movements are executed. It is not less so when very hot, or quite cold. It is wrong to enter the water in a perspira-tion, however trifling it may be. After violent exercises, it is better to wash and employ friction than to bathe. Persons of plethoric temperament, who are subject to periodical evacuations, such as haemorrhoids, or even to cutaneous eruptions, will do well to abstain from swimming during the appearance of these afflictions.

Dress

Every swimmer should use short drawers, and might, in particular places, use canvas slippers. It is even of great im-portance to be able to swim in jacket and trousers.

Aids

The aid of the hand is much preferable to corks or blad-ders, because it can be withdrawn gradually and insensibly. With this view, a grown-up person may take the learner in his arms, carry him into the water breast high, place him nearly flat upon it, support him by one hand under the breast, and direct him as to attitude and action. If the sup-port of the hand be very gradually withdrawn, the swimmer will, in the course of the first ten days, find it quite unneces-sary. When the aid of the hand cannot be obtained, inflated membranes or corks may be employed. The only argument for their use is, that attitude and action may be perfected while the body is thus supported; and that, with some contrivance, they also may gradually be laid aside, though by no means so easily as the hand.

The best mode of employing corks is to choose a piece about a foot long, and six or seven inches broad; to fasten a band across the middle of it; to place it on the back, so that the upper end may come between the shoulder-blades, where the edge may be rounded; and to tie the band over the breast. Over this, several other pieces of cork, each smaller than the preceding, may be fixed, so that, as the swimmer improves, he may leave them off one by one. Even with all these aids, the young swimmer should never venture out of his depth, if he cannot swim without them.

Cramp

As to cramp, those chiefly are liable to it who plunge into the water when they are heated, who remain in it till they are benumbed with cold, or who exhaust themselves by violent exercise. Persons subject to this affliction must be careful with regard to the selection of the place where they bathe, if they are not sufficiently skilful in swimming to vary their attitudes, and dispense instantly with the use of the limb attacked by cramp. Even when this does occur, the skilful swimmer knows how to reach the shore by the aid of the limbs which are unaffected, while the uninstructed one is liable to be drowned.

If attacked in this way in the leg, the swimmer must strike out the limb with all his strength, thrusting the heel downward and drawing the toes upward, notwithstanding the momentary pain it may occasion; or he may immediately

turn flat on his back, and jerk out the affected limb in the
air, taking care not to elevate it so high as greatly to disturb the balance of the body. If this does not succeed, he
must paddle ashore with his hands, or keep himself afloat
by their aid, until assistance can reach him. Should he even
be unable to float on his back, he must put himself in the
upright position, and keep his head above the surface by
merely striking the water downward with his hands at the
hips, without any assistance from the legs.

PROCEDURE WHEN IN THE WATER, AND USUAL MODE OF FRONT SWIMMING

Entering the Water

Instructors should never force young swimmers to leap
into the water reluctantly. It would be advisable for delic-
ate persons, especially when they intend to plunge in, to
put a little cotton steeped in oil, and afterwards pressed,
in their ears, before entering the water. This precaution
will prevent irritation of the organ of hearing. In entering,
the head should be wetted first, either by plunging in head
foremost, or by pouring water on it, in order to prevent
the pressure of the water driving up the blood into the
head too quickly, and increasing congestion. The swimmer
should next advance, by a clear shelving shore or bank,
where he has ascertained the depth by plumbing or otherwise, till the water reaches his breast; should turn towards
the place of entrance; and, having inflated his breast, lay
it upon the water, suffering that to rise to his chin, the lips
being closed.

Buoyancy in the Water

The head alone is specifically heavier than salt water. Even the legs and arms are specifically lighter; and the trunk is still more so. Thus the body cannot sink in salt water, even if the lungs were filled, except owing to the excessive specific gravity of the head.

Not only the head, but the legs and arms, are specifically heavier than fresh water; but still the hollowness of the trunk renders the body altogether too light to sink wholly under water, so that some part remains above until the lungs become filled. In general, when the human body is immersed, one-eleventh of its weight remains above the surface in fresh water, and one-tenth in salt water.

In salt water, therefore, a person throwing himself on his back, and extending his arms, may easily lie so as to keep his mouth and nostrils free for breathing; and, by a small motion of the hand, may prevent turning, if he perceive any tendency to it. In fresh water, a man cannot long continue in that situation, except by the action of his hands; and if no such action be employed, the legs and lower part of the body will gradually sink into an upright position, the hollow of the breast keeping the head uppermost. If, however, in this position, the head be kept upright above the shoulders, as in standing on the ground, the immersion, owing to the weight of the part of the head out of the water, will reach above the mouth and nostrils, perhaps a little above the eyes. On the contrary, in the same position, if the head be leaned back, so that the face is turned upward, the back part of the head has its weight supported by the water, and the face will rise an inch higher at every inspiration, and will sink as much at every expiration, but never so low that the water can come over the mouth.

For all these reasons, though the impetus given by the fall of the body into water occasions its sinking to a depth proportioned to the force of the descent, its natural buoyancy soon impels it again to the surface, where, after a few oscillations up and down, it settles with the head free.

Unfortunately, ignorant people stretch the arms out to grasp at anything or nothing, and thereby keep the head under; for the arms and head, together exceeding in weight one-tenth of the body, cannot remain above the surface at the same time. The buoyancy of the trunk, then and then only, occasions the head and shoulders to sink, the ridge of the bent back becoming the portion exposed; and, in this attitude, water is swallowed, by which the specific gravity is increased, and the body settles to the bottom. It is, therefore, most important to the safety of the inexperienced to be firmly convinced that the body naturally floats.

To satisfy the beginner of the truth of this, Dr Franklin advises him to choose a place where clear water deepens gradually, to walk into it till it is up to his breast, to turn his face to the shore, and to throw an egg into the water between him and it – so deep that he cannot fetch it up but by diving. To encourage him to take it up, he must reflect that his progress will be from deep to shallow water, and that at any time he may, by bringing his legs under him, and standing on the bottom, raise his head far above the water. He must then plunge under it, having his eyes open, before as well as after going under; throw himself towards the egg, and endeavour, by the action of his hands and feet against the water, to get forward till within reach of it. In this attempt, he will find that the water brings him up against his inclination, that it is not so easy to sink as he imagined, and that he cannot, but by force, get down to the egg. Thus he feels the power of water to support him, and learns to confide in that power; while his endeavours to overcome it, and reach the egg, teach him the manner of acting on the water with his feet and hands, as he afterwards must in swimming, in order to support his head higher above the water, or to go forward through it.

If, then, any person, however unacquainted with swimming, will hold himself perfectly still and upright, as if standing with his head somewhat thrown back so as to rest on the surface, his face will remain above the water, and he will enjoy full freedom of breathing. To do this most effectually, the head must be so far thrown back that the chin is higher than the forehead, the breast inflated, the back quite hollow, and the hands and arms kept under water. If these directions be carefully observed, the face will float above the water, and the body will settle in a diagonal direction (Plate XXIII. *fig.* 1).

In this case, the only difficulty is to preserve the balance of the body. This is secured, as described by Bernardi, by extending the arms laterally under the surface of the water, with the legs separated, the one to the front and the other behind: thus presenting resistance to any tendency of the body to incline to either side, forward or backward. This posture may be preserved any length of time (Plate XXIII. *fig.* 2).

The Abbé Paul Moccia, who lived in Naples in 1760, perceived, at the age of fifty, that he could never entirely cover himself in the water. He weighed three hundred pounds

PLATE XXIII

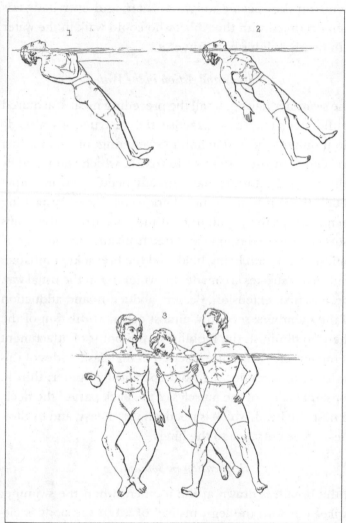

(Italian weight), but being very fat, he lost at least thirty pounds in the water. Robertson had just made his experiments on the specific weight of man; and everybody was then occupied with the Abbé, who could walk in the water with nearly half his body out of it.

Attitude and Action in the Water

The swimmer having, by all the preceding means, acquired confidence, may now practise the instructions already given on attitude and action in swimming: or he may first proceed with the system of Bernardi, which immediately follows. As the former have already been given in ample detail, there is nothing new here to be added respecting them, except that, while the attitude is correct, the limbs must be exercised calmly, and free from all hurry and trepidation, the breath being held, and the breast kept inflated, while a few strokes are made. In swimming in the usual way, there is, first, extension, flexion, abduction and adduction of the members; secondly, almost constant dilation of the chest, to diminish the mobility of the point of attachment of the muscles which are inserted in the elastic sides of this cavity, and to render the body specifically lighter; thirdly, constant action of the muscles of the back part of the neck, to raise the head, which is relatively very heavy, and to allow the air free entrance to the lungs.

Respiration in Swimming

If the breath is drawn at the moment when the swimmer strikes out with the legs, instead of when the body is elevated by the hands descending towards the hips, the head partially sinks, the face is driven against the water, and the mouth becomes filled. If, on the contrary, the breath is drawn when the body is elevated by the hands descending towards the hips (when the progress of the body forward consequently ceases, and when the face is no longer driven against the water, but is elevated above the surface) then, not only cannot the water enter, but if the mouth were at other times even with, or partly under the surface, no water could enter it, as the air, at such times, driven outward between the lips, would effectually prevent it. The breath should accordingly be expired while the body, at the next stroke, is sent forward by the action of the legs.

Coming out of the Water

Too much fatigue in the water weakens the strength and presence of mind necessary to avoid accidents. A person who is fatigued, and remains there without motion, soon becomes weak and chilly. As soon as he feels fatigued, chill, or numb, he should quit the water, and dry and dress himself as quickly as possible. Friction, previous to dressing, drives the blood over every part of the body, creates an agreeable glow, and strengthens the joints and muscles.

UPRIGHT SWIMMING

Bernardi's System

The principal reasons given by Bernardi for recommending the upright position in swimming are: its conformity to the accustomed movement of the limbs; the freedom it gives to the hands and arms, by which any impediment may be removed, or any offered aid readily laid hold of; vision all round; a much greater facility of breathing; and lastly, that much less of the body is exposed to the risk of being laid hold of by persons struggling in the water.

The less we alter our method of advancing in the water from what is habitual to us on shore, the more easy do we find a continued exercise of it. The most important consequence of this is that, though a person swimming in an upright posture advances more slowly, he is able to continue his course much longer; and certainly nothing can be more beneficial to a swimmer than whatever tends to husband his strength, and to enable him to remain long in the water with safety.

Bernardi's primary object is to enable the pupil to float in an upright posture, and to feel confidence in the buoyancy of his body. He accordingly supports the pupil under the shoulders until he floats tranquilly with the head and part of the neck above the surface, the arms being stretched out horizontally under water. From time to time, the supporting arm is removed, but again restored, so as never to suffer the head to sink, which would disturb the growing confidence, and give rise to efforts destructive of the success of the lesson. In this early stage, the unsteadiness of the body is the chief difficulty to be overcome.

The head is the great regulator of our movements in water. Its smallest inclination to either side instantly operates on the whole body; and, if not corrected, throws it into a horizontal posture. The pupil must, therefore, restore any disturbance of equilibrium by a cautious movement of the head alone in an opposite direction. This first lesson being familiarized by practice, he is taught the use of the legs and arms for balancing the body in the water. One leg being stretched forward, the other backward, and the arms laterally, he soon finds himself steadily sustained, and independent of further aid in floating.

When these first steps have been gained, the sweeping semicircular motion of the arms is shown. This is practised slowly, without motion forward, until attained with precision. After this, a slight inclination of the body from the upright position occasions its advancing. The motion of striking with the legs is added in the same measured manner; so that the pupil is not perplexed by the acquisition of more than one thing at a time. In this method, the motions of both arms and legs differ from those we have so carefully described, only in so far as they are modified by a more upright position. It is optional, therefore, with the reader, to practise either method. The general principles of both are now before him.

The upright position a little inclined backward (which, like every other change of posture, must be done deliberately, by the corresponding movement of the head), reversing in this case the motion of the arms, and striking the flat part of the foot down and a little forward, gives the motion backward, which is performed with greater ease than when the body is laid horizontally on the back. According to this system, Bernardi says, a swimmer ought, at every stroke, to urge himself forward a distance equal to the length of his body. A good swimmer ought to make about three miles an hour. A good day's journey may thus be achieved, if the strength be used with due discretion, and the swimmer be familiar with the various means by which it may be recruited.

Of Bernardi's successful practice, he says:

> Having been appointed to instruct the youths of the
> Royal Naval Academy of Naples in the art of swimming,
> a trial of the proficiency of the pupils took place, under
> the inspection of a number of people assembled on
> the shore for that purpose, on the tenth day of their
> instruction. A twelve-oared boat attended the progress
> of the pupils, from motives of precaution. They swam
> so far out in the bay, that at length the heads of the
> young men could with difficulty be discerned with
> the naked eye; and the Major-General of Marine,
> Forteguerri, for whose inspection the exhibition was
> intended, expressed serious apprehensions for their
> safety. Upon their return to the shore, the young men,
> however, assured him that they felt so little exhausted
> as to be willing immediately to repeat the exertion.

An official report on the subject has also been drawn up by
commission (appointed by the Neapolitan government),
after devoting a month to the investigation of Bernardi's
plan; and it states as follows:

> Firstly, It has been established by the experience of more
> than a hundred persons of different bodily constitutions,
> that the human body is lighter than water, and conse-
> quently will float by nature; but that the art of swimming
> must be acquired, to render that privilege useful.
>
> Secondly, That Bernardi's system is new, in so far
> as it is founded on the principle of husbanding the
> strength, and rendering the power of recruiting it easy.
> The speed, according to the new method, is no doubt

diminished; but security is much more important than speed; and the new plan is not exclusive of the old, when occasions require great effort.

Thirdly, That the new method is sooner learnt than the old, to the extent of advancing a pupil in one day as far as a month's instruction on the old plan.

Treading Water

This differs little from the system just described. In it, the position is upright; but progression is obtained by the action of the legs alone. There is little power in this method of swimming: but it may be very useful in rescuing drowning persons.

The arms should be folded across, below the breast, or compressed against the hips, and the legs employed as in front swimming, except as to time and extent. They should perform their action in half the usual time, or two strokes should be taken in the time of one; because, acting perpendicularly, each stroke would otherwise raise the swimmer too much, and he would sink too low between the strokes, were they not quickly to follow each other. They should also work in about two-thirds of the usual space, preserving the upper or stronger, and omitting the lower or weaker, part of the stroke.

There is, however, another mode of treading water, in which the thighs are separated, and the legs slightly bent, or curved together, as in a half-sitting posture. Here the legs are used alternately, so that, while one remains more contracted, the other, less so, describes a circle. By this method, the swimmer does not seem to hop in the water, but remains nearly at the same height. Plate XXIII. *fig.* 3

represents both these methods, and shows their peculiar adaptation to relieve drowning persons.

BACK SWIMMING

In swimming on the back, the action of the thoracic members is weaker, because the swimmer can support himself on the water without their assistance. The muscular contractions take place principally in the muscles of the abdominal members, and in those of the anterior part of the neck. Though little calculated for progression, it is the easiest of all methods, because, much of the head being immersed, little effort is required for support. For this purpose, the swimmer must lie down gently upon the water; the body extended; the head kept in a line with it, so that the back and much of the upper part of the head may be immersed; the head and breast must remain perfectly unagitated by the action of the legs; the hand laid on the thighs (Plate XXIV. *fig*. 1) and the legs employed as in front swimming, care being taken that the knees do not rise out of the water (Plate XXIV. *fig*. 2). The arms may, however, be used in various ways in swimming on the back.

In the method called winging, the arms are extended till in a line with each other; they must then be struck down to the thighs, with the palms turned in that direction, and the thumbs inclining downward to increase the buoyancy (Plate XXIV. *fig*. 3); the palms must then be moved edgewise, and the arms elevated as before (Plate XXIV. *fig*. 4), and so on, repeating the same actions. The legs should throughout make one stroke as the arms are struck down, and another as they are elevated. The other mode, called finning, differs from this only in the stroke of the arms being shorter, and made in the same time as that of the legs.

In back swimming, the body should be extended after each stroke, and long pauses made between these. The act of passing from front to back, or back to front swimming, must always be performed immediately after throwing out the feet. To turn from the breast to the back, the legs must be raised forward, and the head thrown backward, until the body is in a right position. To turn from the back to the breast, the legs must be dropped, and the body thrown forward on the breast.

FLOATING

Floating is properly a transition from swimming on the back. To effect it, it is necessary, while the legs are gently exercising, to extend the arms as far as possible beyond the head, equidistant from, and parallel with, its sides, but never rising above the surface; to immerse the head rather deeply, and elevate the chin more than the forehead; to inflate the chest while taking this position, and so to keep it as much as possible; and to cease the action of the legs, and put the feet together (Plate XXV. *fig.* 1). The swimmer will thus be able to float, rising a little with every inspiration, and falling with every expiration. Should the feet descend, the loins may be hollowed.

SIDE SWIMMING

For this purpose, the body may be turned either upon the right or left side: the feet must perform their usual motions:

PLATE XXIV

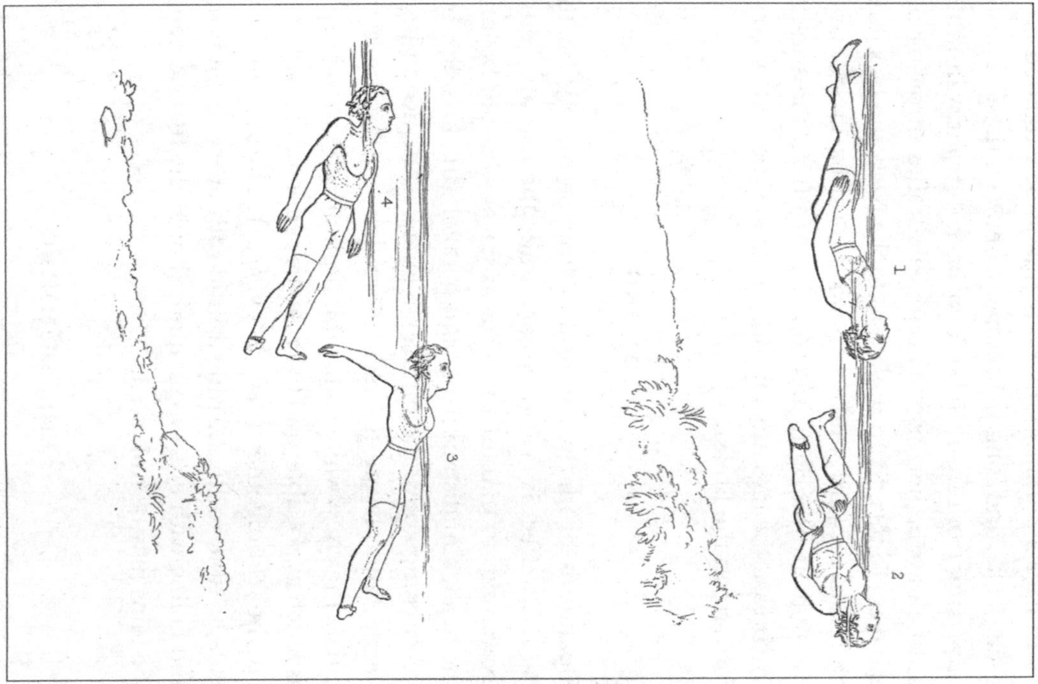

PLATE XXV

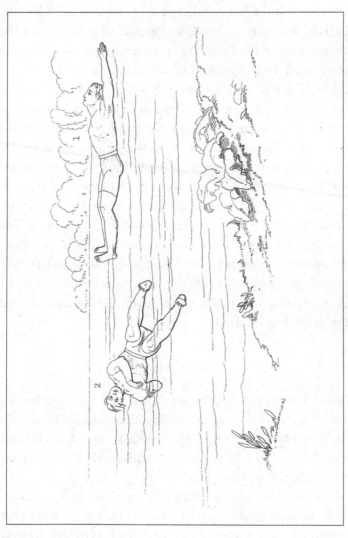

SIDE SWIMMING   FLOATING

the arms also require peculiar guidance. In lowering the left, and elevating the right side, the swimmer must strike forward with the left hand, and sideways with the right; the back of the latter being front instead of upward, and the thumb side of the hand downward to serve as an oar. In turning on the right side, the swimmer must strike out with the right hand, and use the left as an oar. In both cases, the lower arm stretches itself out quickly, at the same time that the feet are striking; and the upper arm strikes at the same time that the feet are impelling, the hand of the latter arm beginning its stroke on a level with the head. While this hand is again brought forward, and the feet are contracted, the lower hand is drawn back towards the breast, rather to sustain than to impel (Plate XXV. *fig.* 2). As side swimming presents to the water a smaller surface than front swimming, it is preferable when rapidity is necessary. But, though generally adopted when it is required to pass over a short distance with rapidity, it is much more fatiguing than the preceding methods.

PLUNGING

In the leap to plunge, the legs must be kept together, the arms close, and the plunge made either with the feet or the head foremost. With the feet foremost, they must be kept together, and the body inclined backward. With the head foremost, the methods vary.

In the deep plunge, which is used where it is known that there is depth of water, the swimmer has his arms outstretched, his knees bent, and his body leant forward (Plate XXVI. *fig.* 1), till the head descends nearly to the feet, when the spine and knees are extended. This plunge may be made without the slightest noise. When the swimmer rises to the surface, he must not open his mouth before previously repelling the water.

In the flat plunge, which is used in shallow water, or where the depth is unknown, and which can be made only from a small height, the swimmer must fling himself forward, in order to extend the line of the plunge as much as possible under the surface of the water; and, as soon as he touches it, he must keep his head up, his back hollow, and his hands stretched forward, flat and inclined upward. He will thus dart forward a considerable way close under the surface, so that his head will reach it before the impulse ceases to operate (Plate XXVI. *fig.* 2).

DIVING

The swimmer may prepare for diving by taking a slow and full inspiration, letting himself sink gently into the water, and expelling the breath by degrees, when the heart begins to beat strongly. In order to descend in diving, the head must be bent forward upon the breast; the back made round; and the legs thrown out with greater vigour than usual; but the arms and hands, instead of being struck forward as in swimming, must move rather backward, or come out lower, and pass more behind (Plate XXVII. *fig.* 1). The eyes should, meanwhile, be kept open, as, if the water be clear, it enables the diver to ascertain its depth, and see whatever lies at the bottom; and, when he has obtained a perpendicular position, he should extend his hands like feelers.

PLATE XXVI

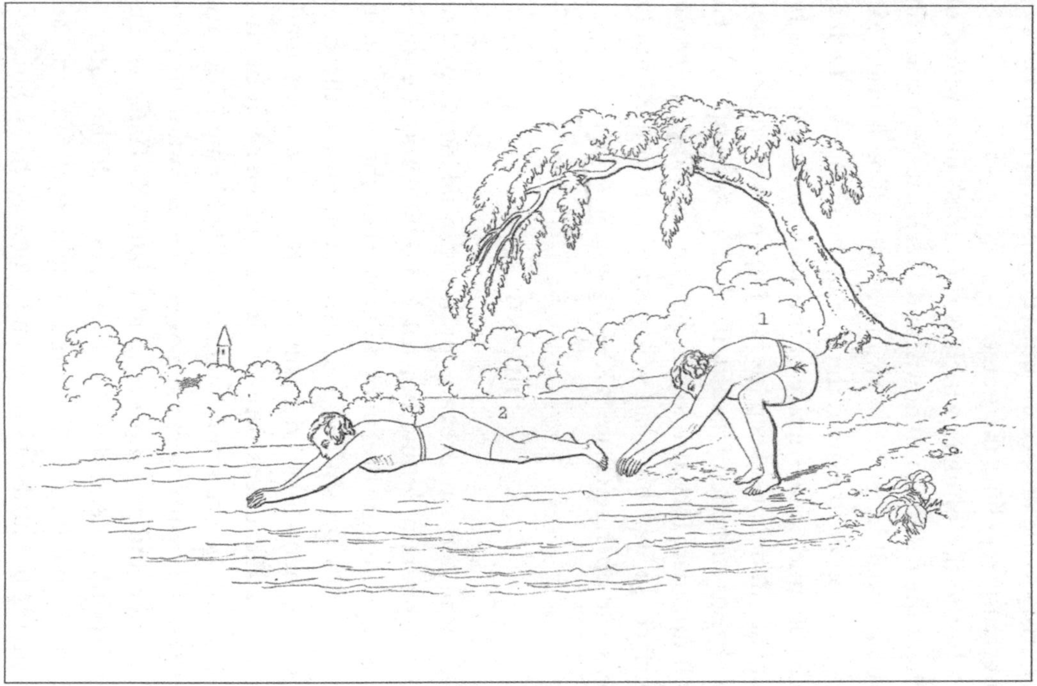

SWIMMING – PLUNGING

PLATE XXVII

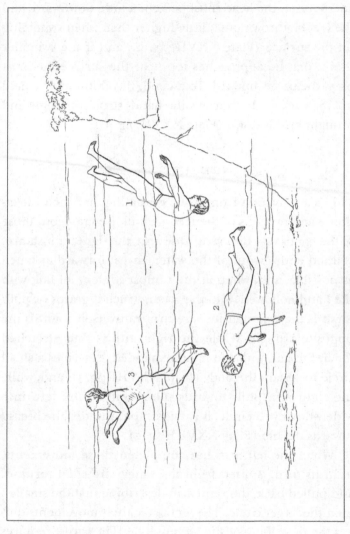

SWIMMING – DIVING

To move forward, the head must be raised, and the
back straightened a little. Still, in swimming between top
and bottom, the head must be kept a little downward, and
the feet be thrown out a little higher than when swimming
on the surface (Plate XXVII. *fig.* 2); and if the swimmer
thinks that he approaches too near the surface, he must
press the palms upward. To ascend, the chin must be held
up, the back made concave, the hands struck out high, and
brought briskly down (Plate XXVII. *fig.* 3).

THRUSTING

This is a transition from front swimming, in which the attitude and motions of the feet are still the same, but those
of the hands very different. One arm, the right for instance,
is lifted entirely out of the water, thrust forward as much
as possible, and, when at the utmost stretch, let fall, with
the hand hollowed, into the water, which it grasps or pulls
towards the swimmer in its return transversely towards the
opposite arm-pit. While the right arm is thus stretched
forth, the left, with the hand expanded, describes a small
circle to sustain the body (Plate XXVIII. *fig.* 1), and, while
the right arm pulls towards the swimmer, the left, in a
widely-described circle, is carried rapidly under the breast,
towards the hip (Plate XXVIII. *fig.* 2).

When the left arm has completed these movements,
it, in its turn, is lifted from the water, stretched forward,
and pulled back, the right arm describing first the smaller,
then the larger circle. The feet make their movements during the describing of the larger circle. The thrust requires
much practice; but, when well acquired, it not only relieves

the swimmer, but enables him to make great advance in the water, and is applicable to cases where rapidity is required for a short distance.

SPRINGING

Some swimmers, at every stroke, raise not only their neck and shoulders, but breast and body, out of the water. This, when habitual, exhausts without any useful purpose. As an occasional effort, however, it may be useful in seizing objects above; and it may then best be performed by the swimmer drawing his feet as close as possible under his body, stretching his hands forward, and, with both feet and hands, striking the water strongly, so as to throw himself out of it as high as the hips.

ONE-ARM SWIMMING

Here the swimmer must be more erect than usual, hold his head more backward, and use the legs and arm more quickly and powerfully. The arm, at its full extent, must be struck out rather across the body, and brought down before, and the breast kept inflated. This mode of swimming is best adapted for assisting persons who are drowning, and should be frequently practised – the learner carrying first under, then over the water, a weight of a few pounds.

In assisting drowning persons, however, great care should be taken to avoid being caught hold of by them. They should be approached from behind, and driven before, or drawn after the swimmer to the shore, by the intervention, if possible, of anything that may be at hand, and if nothing

PLATE XXVIII

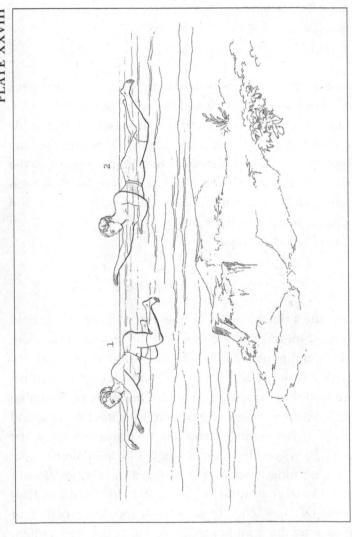

SWIMMING – THRUSTING

be at hand, by means of their hair; and they should, if possible, be got on their backs. Should they attempt to seize the swimmer, he must cast them loose immediately; and, if seized, drop them to the bottom, from whence they will endeavour to rise to the surface.

Two swimmers treading water may assist a drowning person by seizing him, one under each arm, and carrying him along with his head above water, and his body and limbs stretched out and motionless.

FEATS IN SWIMMING

Men have been known to swim in their clothes a distance of 4,000 feet.

Others have performed 2,200 feet in twenty-nine minutes.

Some learn to dive and bring out of the water burdens as heavy as a man.[2]

FINIS

---

2. This art, however, has made little if any progress from the earliest records that we possess of it. Leander's feat of passing from Abydos to Sestos, was the crack performance of antiquity; and it was the ultra achievement of Lord Byron, probably one of the best swimmers of our day. – ED. Fifth Edition.

And for sedentary ladies, you might consider . . .

WALKER'S EXERCISES
FOR LADIES

CALCULATED TO

PRESERVE AND IMPROVE BEAUTY

AND

TO PREVENT AND CORRECT PERSONAL DEFECTS
inseparable from constrained or careless habits

FOUNDED ON

Physiological Principles

BY DONALD WALKER

PECULIARITIES OF THE PRESENT SYSTEM

IT is universally complained that the exercises for ladies at present taught are in many instances frivolous, in other instances severe, in all destitute of system; and the employment of soldiers to teach young ladies to walk, a practice adopted by many parents and heads of seminaries, is generally deprecated.

The military principles of exercise are in most instances excellent; but the stiffness acquired under the practical tuition of sergeants and corporals, is justly observed to be 'adverse to all the principles of grace, and destructive of that buoyant lightness which is so conducive to ease and elegance in the young.'

It is my wish here to combine whatever is really good in the military principles, and in the exercises for ladies as at present taught, to reject what is injurious, to add what seems equally new and necessary, and to present a system suited to the female constitution, nature, and character.

Of the exercises which I here recommend, none accordingly require more strength than the young female possesses, none entail the slightest inconvenience, and all, while they best bestow health, strength, and activity, are calculated to preserve grace and beauty. The whole, I trust, are well suited to the development of the physical faculties in young females, without injury to the perfection of the moral ones.

The introductory views which I give of the structure of the body as connected with exercise – of its functions as affected by exercise; of the constraint to which it is wrongly subjected; of the debility which this causes; of the wrong positions which result from this debility and from the particular pursuits of education when ill directed; of the deformity in which these terminate; of the injury to health and to intellect which accompanies this; and of the particular and special utility of exercises – these views will be acceptable to every parent who desires to know the reasoning by which is guided the education of those who are dearest to him.

The particular exercises, as already said, equally reject whatever is frivolous and whatever is severe, retaining all that contributes to health, strength, beauty of form, and grace of motion.

To obtain the correct position of the figure, the military position of the whole figure,[1] the positions for the feet in dancing, the military extensions for the arms, and the Spanish exercise, are given.

To increase the power and freedom of the arms, the use of dumb-bells, and, which is far more valuable, that of

1. The military principles and practices are duly appreciated throughout this work, as those found by the most extensive experience on the most unfavourable subjects, to be upon the whole the best calculated to prevent or remedy every tendency to deformity.

the Indian sceptres, is described – the latter deriving its name from the form of the instrument which ladies employ, instead of the Indian Clubs used by men. A few of the simplest and most elementary of these exercises are now taught to soldiers for the same purpose for which they are here given: all the more graceful ones are here for the first time added for ladies. The latter will be found to be by far the most useful and most beautiful exercises that ever were introduced into physical education; having vast advantages over the dumb-bells in both these respects, and rendering indeed all other exercises for the arms quite useless. *Of these beautiful exercises, both the more simple military ones, and the more advanced and graceful ones now added, are here for the first time described in any work.*

To improve the lower limbs, the position in walking, the balance step, the mechanism of walking in all the paces, and various exercises for the feet, are described; the art of walking well being particularly attended to, *and more accurately described than usual.*

Observations on dancing are subjoined; a series of remarks on deportment, &c. are added; and games of exercise are noticed.

Lastly, the appropriation and guidance of exercises are discussed.